Communication
Manager's

Annie Phillips

Independent Health Advisor
Management Consultant to General Practice

Radcliffe Medical Press

Radcliffe Medical Press Ltd
18 Marcham Road
Abingdon
Oxon OX14 1AA
United Kingdom

www.radcliffe-oxford.com
The Radcliffe Medical Press electronic catalogue and online ordering facility.
Direct sales to anywhere in the world.

British Library Cataloguing in Publication Data

A catalogue record for this book is available from the British Library.

ISBN 1 85775 534 0

Typeset by Advance Typesetting Ltd, Oxfordshire
Printed and bound by TJ International Ltd, Padstow, Cornwall

Contents

Foreword

In this book Annie Phillips takes a comprehensive look at ways of improving communication and management in general practice. She identifies the skills required of a practice manager and as any reader working in general practice knows, the job is more complex than that of the average manager working in the commercial world. It involves taking responsibility for not just one aspect of the business – for that is what general practice has become – but for everything, the finances, the premises, the staff, effective use of information technology and liaison with other health professionals locally and regionally.

There are many sound management practices described in this book that should help anyone trying to cope with the complexities of practice management. The author poses questions and sets exercises throughout the book that provide the reader with an opportunity to check the relevance of certain topics to their own particular experience.

In the chapter on team leadership, Annie Phillips mentions Belbin, quoted in most books on management, for his theory of the different types of people required to constitute an effective team. Having read this book, practice managers will no doubt be reminded when employing staff that effective teams are usually made up of complementary types of people, rather than similar ones. At least the word 'plant' should evoke thoughts of 'creative innovator' rather than 'garden organism' in future.

This book should be on the shelf in every practice, serving as a handy reference point for managers when undertaking staff appraisal, mediating in partnership disputes or improving communication between staff and patients.

Lyn Longridge
November 2001

About the author

Annie Phillips has written professionally about health and health management since she qualified as a speech and language therapist in 1978. She has over 20 years' NHS experience in primary and secondary care as a clinician and manager.

Her 10 years as a speech and language therapist led to the research and publication of an international dysphasia/dementia screening test, presented at the 1986 British Aphasiology Conference. She has won various prizes and awards for her subsequent work, and in the 1990s she was a finalist in the *Medeconomics'* Good Management Awards, and regional winner in a national British Institute of Management competition on change management.

She worked as a practice and fund manager for a five-partner training practice in central Brighton from 1989 to 1998; from then as an independent health advisor, trainer, and management consultant to general practice.

Throughout her career she has written extensively for the therapy, GP and management press. She currently writes on contemporary management issues for a range of publications, including the *Health Service Journal*, *Community Care*, *Doctor*, *Primary Care Manager* and Croner Publications, with a focus on healthcare politics and human resource management.

As a management consultant, her interest is in organisational analysis and the development of healthy organisations, with a focus on finding ways to manage stresses and conflicts, understanding and alleviating dysfunctional communication and developing effective management strategies.

Annie can be contacted via aphillips@cwcom.net or www.anniephillips.co.uk.

Acknowledgements

Thanks to Bob Sang from the King's Fund, who supported a Learning Set that I was part of in the late 1990s. Bob was an inspirational facilitator and tutor, who prompted the idea for including Chapter 11 in this book.

Thanks also to all the David Salomans Centre tutors, especially Nigel Armstrong and Vivien Martin, for the material on learning and facilitation, and for inspiring me to find out more about organisational processes.

Special thanks to Madeleine Price, my Editor at *Primary Care Management* magazine, for her support and encouragement of my writing over the years, and to those whose friendship and ideas have sustained me, including the East Sussex Fund Manager contingent.

I would like to thank all those whose work I have quoted and acknowledged in the text. My apologies if I have misquoted anyone unintentionally. Every attempt has been made to acknowledge sources. If any queries, errors or omissions are noted, please contact the publisher.

Finally, as always, my very special thanks go to Lin and Chris for allowing me the time out from family life to continue writing.

Part one
A broad look at communication

CHAPTER 1

The foundations of good communication

What are communication skills and why is it important to learn about them? We know that communication skills involve:

- words (written or spoken)
- gestures (body language)
- delivery (tone of voice, pitch, timing)
- symbols
- listening.

Understanding communication is important, as the ability to communicate well is directly related to our ability to be successful – our happiness, relationships and personal growth all depend on effective communication. Good communication is especially important for those in leadership positions as it assists them to:

- make discoveries about themselves and others
- solve problems and develop new skills
- manage conflict, emotion and anger
- understand other people and how they communicate
- self-manage, question their position, adapt, change and grow.

Others appreciate the listening ability, clarity, and honesty of good communicators. Communication is a two-way process which involves sharing information. It is essential for getting along with others and getting things done.

This book's aim is to take those managing within primary care through all these functions. The aim is to improve and enhance the reader's interpersonal communication skills so that they become more effective listeners, responding skillfully and sensitively to the challenges modern healthcare presents us with.

The biggest complaint in general practice is poor communication. To avoid this, those holding leadership responsibilities need to be multi-skilled. To be an effective team leader, you need to share ideas, concerns, suggestions and other information with those on your team, your superiors, and people out-side your organisation. You may need to:

- give work assignments or instructions
- make or discuss changes in procedures
- respond to enquiries
- tell people how they are doing
- solicit ideas, thoughts or information.

The interpersonal communication skills needed in management are wide-based, functional or process-orientated and include such things as:

- motivating/leading/listening/instructing/organising
- writing/presenting/chairing/counselling
- facilitating/supervising/delegating/interviewing/appraising.

Each process has its own skill, and each skill can be learnt. Communication is complex. It involves:

- a message: statements, questions, commands or warnings
- a language: words, symbols and gestures make up the elements of language
- a system: communication occurs through touch, silence, voice, gestures, writing.

The way something is communicated – its delivery – tells us a lot about the content. Facial expressions, such as smiles and frowns, play a part in com-munication, as do:

- timing and speed: communication is affected when people talk too quickly, cut one another off, or wait too long to bring up an issue
- body language: clenched fists, eye contact, head position
- word choice: will tell us if the situation is public or private, doubtful or hopeful, formal or informal, serious or relaxed
- tone of voice: feelings such as sorrow, pride, anger, impatience, can all be expressed.

Words and symbols have different meanings among different cultures. Humour may help or hinder; gestures can be misinterpreted. We can never assume our communication is understood or accepted by others; good communicators check they have been understood.

Why is communication so important?

Many of those working in healthcare have lost sight of the importance of communication – there is so much to do, and so little time to accomplish what is needed. When stretched, it seems quicker and easier to get on with a job, and keeping people informed feels difficult because there is so much to do and tell.

Those leading in healthcare need to make a commitment to employee communication. Not to inform is to patronise – if we assume the staff do not need to know, they will feel undervalued and disrespected. Communication has to be two-way – all employees have views, good ideas or suggestions on alternative ways of working; just ask and be prepared to listen. Other people often have a clear outside vision on a project, whereas those working daily on the practicalities and details may lose sight of its simplicity. Managers and GPs do not always have the answers. Of course, if we accept that visibility and openness are important, we need to recognise that mistakes will be aired in the same way as triumphs.

The process of communication

Consider some of the functions of communication in more detail. Communication is multi-directional – it can be impersonal, often written, directional and one-way.

- It can be face-to-face.
- It can be outward – towards the patients or external organisations such as the employing trust.
- It can also go 'up' from employees to employer.
- It may go sideways – if you utilise team work.
- It may go 'down' from employer to employee.

To communicate successfully people need skills which can be learned or applied. Different types of meeting, for example, have different functions. Each one may utilise a different set of skills – chairing, facilitating, presenting, team-building, instructing, etc.

Communication may be defined as 'the exchange of information between a sender and a receiver with the inference of meaning'. Thus an individual's personality, history, motivation and personal development all affect the way s/he hears, or receives, information transmitted by another – these all affect communication accuracy. Some other less visible factors also have a big influence.

- Organisational structure.
- Interpersonal relationships.
- Incomplete information.

Organisational structure

Communication is a central organisational process. The exchange of information between different participants links the various subsystems of the organisation, and builds and reinforces interdependence between them.

General practice is hierarchical, with superiors (the medics) and subordinates (the staff). This arrangement can create communication difficulties, with the lower status members – those without much power – suppressing unfavourable information because they worry that their superiors may regard them unfavourably if they pass on negative material. Thus, less powerful members only communicate what they feel you want to hear. Depending where you fit into this hierarchy, you may or may not be party to these negative comments. If you are a manager who sees the partners as your peers, you will feel happier passing on 'bad' news to them. However, you then may not hear all you need to from your subordinates. On the other hand, if you stand with the staff, and represent their voice, you may find it difficult to stand your ground with the doctors. A skilled communicator will fit somewhere between, and gain respect from both.

The larger and more specialised your work groups are within your organisation, the greater the possibilities for misunderstanding, as the employees in different teams have access to more, and very different, information. This discourages sharing and increases the potential for misunderstandings. Differences in power, goals and expertise between departments (finance, personnel, secretarial, reception, management, nursing) may make communication difficult and give room for discord, gossip and backbiting to flourish.

Interpersonal relationships

The relationship between the two people communicating also affects the accuracy with which messages are given and received. An important factor in this is how much **trust** there is between the two – when people trust each other communication tends to be more accurate and open. When the receiver of the message has considerable **influence** over the sender, the communication may be modified or guarded – it would make sense that someone seeking promotion would modify their message in a way that enhances their position or personal development. **Group norms**, or expected standards of behaviour, may limit the amount or type of information people feel they can legitimately discuss. The type and content of communication also differs in different contexts – the relaxed chat of the staff room differs from the more formal discussion in meetings.

Incomplete information

This is particularly relevant when an employee's performance is being appraised or discussed. If relying on only one source of information when judging performance, persistent biases are likely to occur.

So, what are some of the barriers to effective communication and how can we make ourselves heard above these?

Barriers to effective communication

Lack of feedback

If we communicate something without any acknowledgement that we have been heard and understood, we cannot assume that our message has been understood. Managers often give large quantities of information and direction without provision or opportunity for their staff to indicate that they have understood. There are various reasons why this happens.

- Lack of trust in the other's ability to contribute.
- Lack of personal confidence ('They might think I don't know the answer').
- An assumption that people have the same goals, ideals and motivations as ourselves ('But it's obvious I meant ...').
- Poor communication skills – where two-way communication is not respected.

Everyone has a responsibility to encourage two-way communication. If the staff fail to inform their boss about their needs and values, or withhold information because they distrust him or her or are antagonistic, the boss has a responsibility to redefine the trust. Communication should be as open as possible, and one way this can be achieved is to create a supportive communication climate where people feel able to talk without feeling judged.

Managers need to avoid the following behaviours:

- *Ridicule, lecturing*: being dismissive, ordering. **Instead**, communicate respectfully.
- *Evaluating*: when we behave defensively we judge – we blame, call for different behaviour, praise. **Instead**, create a supportive environment by giving and asking for information – behave more neutrally.
- *Controlling*: when we attempt to persuade others by imposing our personal attitudes on them. **Instead**, collaborate with your colleague by jointly defining and solving the problem.
- *Strategic communication*: when we attempt to manipulate others. **Instead**, deal with them more spontaneously, openly and without deception.
- *Uncaring behaviour*. **Instead**, demonstrate your concern, show empathy by identifying with your colleague's position.
- *Superiority*. **Instead**, show your respect for others by de-emphasising the status and power differences.
- *Certainty*: being dogmatic, wanting to win rather than solve the problem. **Instead**, show your openness to new information and interpretations, postpone taking sides.

Noise

Interference that occurs during the communication process ('noise') may be audible or inaudible. The presence of a silent third party during a conversation may act as noise in that it distracts the receiver from hearing what the speaker says. The receiver's pre-occupation with an unrelated problem can have the same effect.

The use of language

The choice of words or language in which a sender encodes a message will influence the quality of communication. Because language is an abstract representation of a phenomenon, there is room for interpretation and distortion of the meaning.

Misunderstandings can arise through using words that are too abstract, too general or too vague. Jargon and technical terms frequently create misunderstanding, as does the use of slang or colloquialisms.

Listening deficiencies

The quality of listening by the receiver may help or hurt communication. Effective communication calls for active listening by individuals. Active listening requires the receiver to listen for the total meaning a person conveys, to try to determine both the content of the message and the feelings underlying it. Active listening also calls for noting all the cues, both verbal and non-verbal, in communication.

Improve your ability to be heard

Healthy organisations seem to be strongly influenced by humanistic psychology, where openness, trust and belief in individual growth are paramount. Build an organisational framework that is humanitarian, where the management style is open, reflective, listening and interested. For this to happen, be prepared to learn how to communicate well. Eighty-five percent of communication is non-verbal, communicated in gestures, facial expression and tone of voice.

> **How do you communicate verbally at work?**
>
> Through writing – memos, reports? Do you communicate in groups? In meetings? On the telephone?
>
> Note down why you think there may be crossed wires in each situation.

In any communication:

- both sides need to be interested and involved
- both sides need to be willing to be open and honest
- both sides need to feel heard and understood
- the atmosphere needs to be comfortable
- even if the talking is difficult, the important things get said.

Conversations have to make a difference. Something useful or satisfying usually happens as a result.

To ensure effective communication:

- devote the time
- share
- keep in regular contact
- be assertive
- be specific
- be clear
- be open
- be prepared to negotiate
- value difference
- own your own thoughts and feelings: use 'I' instead of 'you', describe your feelings instead of the other person's behaviour, e.g. 'I feel angry because I don't like having to start all over again' instead of 'I feel angry when you are late'
- respect and recognise feelings
- don't assume
- repeat the message if misunderstood
- compromise if it is reasonable to do so

Table 1.1[1]

Good communication	Poor communication
Working together in partnership	Scoring points to win
Co-operating, nurturing	Being competitive
Making feelings clear	Hiding feelings, being defensive
Explaining needs	Applying pressure, bullying
Sharing the airtime	Dominating the airtime
Responding sensitively	Showing insensitive behaviour
Understanding everyone has a different inner world, and different motivations and experiences	Wanting everyone to be like you, making assumptions
Understanding why the conversation is taking place	Misunderstanding why the conversation is taking place
Being open to anything	Attacking or being threatening
Being interested by difference	Patronising or putting down
Listening and watching	Ignoring, not paying attention
Advising and supporting	Lecturing, being critical or judgemental
Knowing yourself, and being true to self	Constructing a false public persona
Valuing your experience	Giving unwanted advice, preaching
Respecting and valuing your views	Trivialising views
Being clear, staying on track	Rambling
Reflecting back to show understanding, responding with interest	Always missing the point
Welcoming difficulties and conflict as opportunities to learn	Avoiding conflict
Checking that it is a good time to talk	Barging in regardless
Being open-minded	Being closed-minded
Balancing questions with talking about self	Asking too many questions, interrogating
Allowing plenty of time	Being impatient
Cutting the tale up into bite-size chunks	Dumping too much information
Giving people the opportunity to respond	Overloading or boring
Encouraging the flow	Avoiding
Prompting	Taking up all the room
Asking	Telling

- listen to the other person
- accept responsibility
- choose the right moment
- summarise
- keep an open mind
- show you understand, and say when you don't
- don't give advice unless asked for
- base any feedback on facts
- sandwich a negative between two positives
- express your feelings
- innovate: take chances and risks
- accept criticism when appropriate

- prompt others to express themselves honestly
- empower yourself
- be yourself.

In summary, good communicators:

- read the situation
- engage attention
- make the meaning clear
- tell the story
- look for clues
- check understanding
- say what is on their mind
- summarise.

Make a note of the good and poor communicators in your practice.

Non-verbal communication

How you dress, the apparent wealth and status reflected in your surroundings, your use of time and space could clarify the meaning of verbal communication or increase its impact.

Non-verbal signals may also contradict a verbal message or alter its meaning. In manager/subordinate communication there are also the obstacles to frank expressions of opinion or full disclosure of information. A good communicator watches out for signs of contradiction or discomfort and encourages a more honest discourse.

If you indicate your authority non-verbally through power dressing or use of office space, you may need to make an effort to meet others more equally. Watch for the non-verbal signs of dominance around the practice – who holds the biggest space, e.g. the largest consulting room; do they have a clear, uncluttered desk and surroundings? A polished wooden desk with only a blotter pad and fountain pen strikes fear in most of us! The higher up the organisation you go, the less you have to **do** (dirty your hands) – your job is only to think.

An insecure manager may place their desk a considerable distance from the door, so whoever comes in has to walk some way before being within communicable distance – a very humbling and humiliating experience. Unless you need to remind your staff you mean business, create a more comfortable, less oppressive, communication environment.

- Sit them at right angles to you, not opposite.
- Do not place a desk between you.

Status should come to you through being respected, not feared.

Watch out to see if the non-verbal messages you are receiving or giving serve to underline or undermine the verbal message. If the latter, try creating a more supportive communication climate to get and give a clearer picture.

Listen actively

Without confusing it with the professional role of counsellor in the practice, many managers and GPs have a first line counselling role. If anyone is distressed, angry or has something of importance to say, your role is to listen.

Good listeners:

- *Listen*: pay close, interested, attention.
- *Paraphrase*: demonstrate they have correctly perceived the sender's inner state and understood, e.g. 'are you saying you dislike that kind of work ...?'
- *Ask questions*: to clarify the position, or reflect back that you have heard, e.g. 'so that made you feel very angry?'
- *Never interrupt*.
- *Never advise* or suggest solutions.
- *Allow feelings*: do not try to stop them, but encourage them – suppressing feelings will only increase the sender's discomfort and discourage them from trusting you.

If people have the chance to talk, uninterrupted and with full attention on them, they usually unravel the problem themselves.

Discriminating language

Take care around the use of offensive language, and challenge it if you hear it. Unwitting prejudice, ignorance, thoughtlessness and stereotyping do nothing but disadvantage those in the minority. This prejudice often extends to discrimination against sexuality, class, disability or culture as well as race.

Certain factors in our society which shift our sense of power in relation to others are shown in Table 1.2.[2]

Table 1.2

Factors which shift power up	Factors which shift power down
Being aged 25–45	Being young or old
Being middle or upper class	Being working class
Being white	Being black or from an ethnic minority
Being English speaking	Having a strong regional accent
Being articulate	Not speaking English well or fluently
Being educated	Being uneducated
Being employed	Being unemployed
Being able bodied	Being disabled in any way
Being tall	Being short
Being attractive	Being ugly
Being a man	Being a woman
Being a professional	Being a victim (of violence or abuse)
Being rich	Being poor
Being average	Being different in any way, through culture, sexuality, having an obvious mental health problem

How can you avoid offending and patronising others?

- What are your feelings about the above?
- What assumptions and attitudes do you already hold?
- Why?
- How might these attitudes impact on other individuals around you?
- However you identify, think about the experience of your opposite number – what would it feel like to be more/less powerful?
- How do you act and behave when faced with your prejudice? Are you dismissive, patronising, hurtful, scared?
- Have you ever used a term that would upset or offend?
- Do you make assumptions about people, for example, assume everyone is heterosexual?
- Have you ever been challenged about your use of language?
- Have you ever responded to a patient in a way that may have deterred or inhibited them from using your services?

Table 1.3 shows some of the negative ways in which certain groups of people can be described. Add your own.

Have you ever examined some of your beliefs and prejudices about your colleagues? Human beings tend to act tribally, we feel safer in groups, and one way we reinforce this feeling of safety is to poke fun at or invalidate the 'other'. Fundamentally, we act through fear and ignorance. What does offensive language tell us about our beliefs? Think about where these attitudes and beliefs have come from. Question those beliefs.

Table 1.3

Area	Preferred term	Instead of
Age	Older people Elderly Over 50s	Old biddy/codger
Gender	Woman Chair	Girl Chairman
Black and ethnic minority communities	Dual heritage Black Asian	Half-caste Coloured Paki
Sexual orientation	Bisexual Lesbian Gay	Bent Poofter

What would it take for you to leave your family, friends and culture and go to a place where you knew no one?

What qualities do you think you would need to do this? List them.

Think again about the question in relation to asylum seekers.

Janet Suzman, actress and civil liberties campaigner, has said that dealing with racism is about having the courage not to let it go unchallenged. Racism lurks just below the surface in so many of us. If we feel we have the permission to say ridiculous things then somebody with a conscience needs to stand up to us – or we to them.

Lateral communication

Once you have perfected the art of communicating upwards and downwards you can then move on to tackling broader communication problems within your organisation, such as team building, leadership and motivating staff. The next chapter will explore the wider processes of communication.

References

1   Bailey A (1997) *Talk Works*, British Communications plc, London.

2   Sourced from *Making it Happen: working towards equality in Cruse Bereavement Care*. Cruse House, 126 Sheen Road, Richmond, Surrey, TW9 1UR. Tel: 020 8939 9530. www.crusebereavementcare.org.uk.

CHAPTER 2

Communication within the practice: practical steps

Policies and procedures

The factors most commonly affecting complaints and clinical negligence claims within the NHS are:[1]

- communication breakdowns
- poor systems and processes
- human error.

Practices need to develop systems to manage clinical and administrative communications, e.g. home visit protocols, tracer systems, complaints procedures. Processes need to be put in place to integrate quality communication into all organisational processes. The basic considerations to avoid communication breakdown across people or systems are to:

- plan ahead
- problem solve
- communicate (keep people involved and informed)
- review and monitor.

Review your systems of communication across the practice.

- Do you create systems to identity and evaluate mistakes?
- Do you share good practice?
- Do you hold regular team meetings?
- Do you have a practice agreement?
- Do you implement and adhere to formal systems?
- Do you educate and provide feedback to staff?

Staff should be informed and consulted about matters likely to affect their employment. Those with a management role in the practice need to create a climate where equity for all and respect for individual differences is ensured. Communication rights should extend across the practice so that staff feel fully and properly trained to do the job they are employed to do, and able to comment or complain to their employers without fear or prejudice.

Impersonal communications

Whenever you write a memo, a newsletter or create a notice for the notice board you create a one-way channel of communication. There are distinct advantages to this – everyone receives the same information, it is clear and unlikely to be misunderstood and it is relatively cheap. The disadvantage is that communication is one-way, so advise people where they can go if they want further information.

Investigate innovative ways of communicating, and keep them current.

- Using video tapes to publicise health promotion activity.
- Rolling electronic message boards for daily changes of information to patients in the waiting room.
- Having local service directories on display – loose-leaf folders detailing local services in the waiting room.

Most practices have administrative protocols, but how many are easily available in a crisis? Write your protocols in a way that is easy to understand by everyone who may need to use them, pilot them, and keep copies in reception, in your office, and with the secretaries.

Tips to reduce communication breakdowns and prevent errors.

- Information should be clear, direct and easy to read.
- Devise procedures for keeping everyone in the practice informed about how it works – especially visiting clinicians and attached staff.
- Write a **locum fact pack** so that all non-principals working in your surgery are familiar with daily and routine practice and referral procedures. Detail any clinical governance requirements, e.g. your mechanisms for recording any adverse incidents.
- Write **induction manuals** so that everyone receives an adequate induction to the job. This includes doctors. A thorough induction will save time in mistakes and questions later on.

See Appendix A for an example induction pack.

Demonstrate good communication habits when giving instructions.

- Ask, don't command.
- Be positive – stress 'what to do' not 'what to avoid'.

- Tell why it is important.
- Requests should leave as much freedom of action as is possible to the receiver, consistent with their ability and training.
- Obtain feedback – don't just assume the person has got the message:
  - ask open-ended questions: 'what do you think?' not 'is that clear?'
  - take the initiative and assume ownership of potential misunderstandings: 'sometimes I'm not sure if I've made myself clear – would you repeat it back to me so I can check myself?'
  - watch for non-verbal signs of doubt or insecurity
  - encourage and reward questions, never punish them.

When you give instructions:

- tell them
- show them
- have them tell you
- have them show you
- have them write it down.

The Transmission Model of Communication.[2]

Where do problems occur? What is missing in this model?

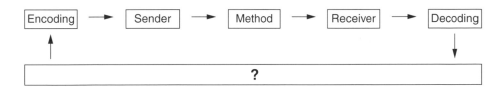

Teach good communication habits. To communicate well in business can bring positive results. Develop good communication habits for writing letters, memos and reports throughout your organisation.

See Appendix B for some suggestions on writing letters, memos and reports.

Formal reports

- Prepare – gather material, select, arrange.
- Use active sentences, e.g. 'Dr S presented a paper' not 'A paper was presented by Dr S'.
- Use concrete nouns.
- Do not make empty assertions, demonstrate using references and quotes.

- Split into paragraphs if too long.
- Seek continuity of thought and fact.
- Avoid verbosity – brevity is a product of good writing.

Administrative considerations

Despite the increase in technology within general practice, paperwork is increasing. More paperwork means more tasks and tighter deadlines. The way paperwork is processed directly affects how smoothly the practice runs.

Forms

Every GP absence involves decisions about surgeries, locums and cancelling appointments, surgeries and clinics. Secretaries, receptionists, nurses and managers all become involved. When designing a form or system to communicate, consider the following.

- Who needs to know?
- How can we ensure they have seen the communication?
- What methods are used to communicate?
- Does the information have to be retained?

Post

Staff and doctors must be able to receive *and* pass on their paperwork easily. Are the following systems organised as well as they could be?

- Staff pigeonholes – by person or department.
- Separate doctor pigeonholes for mail, clinical mail, messages, insurance reports, medical records.
- Incoming mail opened, stamped and sorted.
- Outgoing mail sealed and franked.
- Records kept of both incoming and outgoing mail.

Problem areas occur when papers are lost, taken home by a doctor, left in their car, or submerged in a pile in the consulting room. When paperwork arrives on a desk:

- is it clear to the recipient what has happened so far or are there scribblings all over the paper?
- is there a deadline and, if so, is this clearly marked?
- does the sheet, with all the scribbles, have to be returned to somebody off site?
- who is to see the paper next?
- what is the urgency for passing on the paper?

- are there any confidentiality issues to consider?
- do you habitually make copies?

Protocols

Re-visit protocols for the following.

- Visits, to ensure DVs are not late or missed.
- Urgent v routine appointments.
- Missed or cancelled appointments.
- Telephone messages/advice/call back procedures.
- Labelling, sending and receiving samples.
- Confirming messages are received and/or acted upon.
- Confidentiality.
- Notifying patients of delays.
- Notifying patients of results.
- Checking outstanding referrals.
- The practice post system.
- Returning patient records.
- Maintaining and repairing medical equipment.

How do you communicate within your practice? Do you:

- circulate special newsletters?
- have weekly surgery bulletins?
- hold away days?
- have regular meetings?
- have networked computers with bulletin boards and an e-mail facility?

To limit losses and avoid breakdowns in communication, make your expected standards explicit, train the staff, and distribute these with all staff contracts.

See Appendix C for examples of expected standards for reception staff.

Keep good records

- Are your Medical Records accurate and reliable?
- Are they stored securely and are they easily accessible ?
- Are the notes summarised?
- Are key data easily accessible and kept separate, e.g. prescribing ?
- Are all contacts' notes, including telephone contacts, kept current?
- Is filing up to date?
- Are records kept of investigations sent off, acted upon, and received?
- What is the system for recording recent deaths, terminal illnesses, and discharges from hospital – is this accessible to all?

Communicating with patients

Patient literature

Keeping patients informed improves communication, assists in managing risk, and supports clinical governance guidelines. This section looks at some of the best ways to keep patients informed about the services you offer. The information may be in the form of a newsletter, leaflets, or on a practice website. However it is presented, it must be updated regularly and written in language appropriate for your target audience. The NHS Plan 1999 asks that practices produce a wider range of information in their leaflets. How could you best inform your patients about the following.

- Your list size?
- Accessibility?
- Performance against NSF standards?
- Number of patients removed from list?
- Names of attached staff, their roles and times of availability?
- Any other services you offer, e.g. counselling service, a visiting social worker?
- Information on minor illnesses and common complaints?
- Addresses and contact numbers for relevant local charities and businesses? Be inclusive not discriminatory.
- A way to tell you if any of the information is out of date, or if there is anything they would like to see added?

Some pointers for managers.

- Ask each key staff group to write their own copy.
- Edit it into your preferred house style.
- The average reading age in this country is around 11-years-old – the level of a tabloid newspaper.

When preparing patient literature:

- use plain English
- translate if required
- use words of one to two syllables
- keep all sentences and paragraphs short
- keep language personal: 'you, we, your baby' instead of 'they, those'
- avoid polysyllabic words/double-negatives/jargon/acronyms
- the aim is to inform not impress – be specific not vague
- repeat key information several times
- use positive language
- plan and test with those you are writing for
- use a large font, and print black on yellow to make it accessible to those with visual impairments.

Table 2.1

Instead of	Try
Our aim for this leaflet is to ...	We aim to ...
Keep you up to date with all of our services	Tell you about our:
	• doctors
	• nurses
	• health visitors
	• counsellor
We hope you will find this information useful when deciding whether to see a doctor – or whether someone else in our team can help you	Point you in the right direction
It is not yet possible to ...	We are trying to ...

Patient surveys

Before you embark on constructing your own survey, find out if your PCT advocates using an established one which includes all the types of questions patients may wish to answer regarding:

- access
- availability
- interpersonal care
- continuity of care
- trust
- referrals
- co-ordination of care outside the practice.

If you do want to devise your own, make certain the questions are:

- relevant
- unambiguous
- asked one at a time
- given simple choices of response
- flowing in a logical order
- in a language that your population understands.

Do not:

- make assumptions
- ask leading or biased questions
- use complex, inappropriate or offensive language
- assume that all answers will be honest.

If your PCT cannot help, consider your selection criteria – have you chosen a relevant sample population? Have you piloted it? Invest in specialist help and use specialist software if needed.

Meetings

Best practice shows us organisations where the decision-making is devolved down, and ideas are fed up. Given the biggest complaint in general practice is poor communication, practices that make good use of meeting time go a long way towards alleviating those problems. Partnership meetings are not usually public events, and in most practices feedback to staff from these meetings is rare, at best haphazard and partial, at worst absent altogether. Develop a mechanism to feed back to the staff following these or external reviews. Staff need to feel included in the major decision-making. Here are some facts about meetings in general practice.

- Most people don't like meetings.
- Meetings are essential to foster good two-way communication.
- Meetings need to be held regularly.
- Partners demonstrate their commitment to their employees through attending meetings.
- Practices must feed back to the staff following meetings where staff have been excluded.
- Staff need to feel included in the major decision-making.

In Table 2.2, note if your meetings are well chaired, organised or not, have good attendance, are held frequently enough, or if there is an absence of an agenda and minutes.

Table 2.2

How often are they held?	Are they managed well?	What are the problems?
Diary meetings		
Informal open meetings		
Whole practice meetings		
Partnership meetings		
Reception meetings		
Audit meetings		
Critical incident meetings		
Clinical meetings		
Computer meetings		
Practice nurse meetings		
Community nurse meetings		
Others		

Do your meetings involve one- or two-way communication? At one-to-one meetings such as an appraisal, the employee does most of the talking and the manager supports, questions, summarises and reviews. However, during team meetings, the workers review their performance together and iron out

problems. Communication is two-way, with the manager directing and inform-
ing and the employees advising, suggesting, and problem solving. Chairing
skills are important here – the communication channels have to be controlled
so that the most talkative staff member does not claim all the space. Everybody
needs encouragement to contribute. Listening skills are important too; here is
a space for people to air their views. Larger meetings may be uni-directional,
as information is passed one way only.

Managing meetings. Well-planned and managed meetings are an organisation's most valuable means of communication – they considerably ease the
task of co-ordinating the activities of large and diverse organisations like the
health service.

- Meetings often contract (or expand) to fill the time allotted. Shorten them.
- Give incentives to stay on target – meet before lunch or late afternoon.
- Review the frequency and duration.
- Use definite times/meetings for discussing routine matters.
- Start and finish on time, and never relay the meeting for latecomers.
- Postpone or delegate topics that need further discussion or research.
- Produce action minutes with name and deadline.
- Only speak if you have a real contribution to make.
- Avoid all meetings that do not run smoothly.
- Delegate housekeeping responsibilities.
- Use a skilled, firm and authoritative chair. Interrupt people who:
    - begin philosophical discussions
    - tell long-winded jokes or anecdotes
    - rehearse or re-play meetings without reference to the agenda or
      minutes.
- Ask 'why are we meeting?' If an agenda cannot be produced, there is no
  meeting.

See Appendix D for a questionnaire on how effectively you manage your
meetings.

Problem meetings. Dr Vivien Martin[3] discusses some common themes
in unproductive meetings, which she attributes to ineffective control of people
and time. She gives some excellent ideas on how to counteract these problems. *See* Section 1, Chapter 4 for more information about recognising group
characters and how their behaviours can disrupt meetings. Diffuse the negative aspects of the following behaviours.

- *If the chair is ignored.* The chair has to demonstrate control of the meeting.
  A fine balance has to be achieved. If you are too passive you are seen to
  have lost control, but if you are too domineering you are seen to have
  wrested control but sacrificed the democratic process.

- *If a member comes up with an obviously incorrect comment.* Your intention is not to humiliate, so try: 'that's one way of looking at it', and then add: 'can we reconcile that with the situation we're discussing here?'
- *If you are asked for your opinion.* Are you being put you on the spot or asked to support a particular view?
  - Never take sides.
  - Avoid solving people's problems for them.
  - Confirm that your view is relatively unimportant compared with that of the rest of the group.
  - Try to determine the reason your opinion was sought: 'let's get some views from the rest of the group'.
- *If someone is openly argumentative.* They could be a habitual heckler, or may be normally good-natured but upset by current events.
  - Keep your own temper firmly in check.
  - Calm the group.
  - Try to find merit in one of the points.
  - Move on to something else.
  - Turn to the group and let them correct or reject the statement.
- *If they are over-talkative.* They could be exceptionally well-informed and anxious to receive recognition for this or simply be naturally garrulous.
  - Never be hostile or sarcastic.
  - Slow them down with some difficult questions.
  - Interrupt with: 'that's an interesting point. Let's see what the rest of the group thinks.'
- *If they are inarticulate.* They may lack the ability to put thoughts into comprehensible words.
  - Don't say: 'what you mean is ...'. Better to say: 'let me summarise that'.
  - Restate the point in clearer language without altering the content.
- *If they won't talk.* Your reaction will depend on the motivation – are they bored, do they feel superior, or are they too timid to contribute?
  - Arouse their interest by asking their opinion.
  - If they are the superior type, ask for their view after indicating the respect held for experience. Take care not to overdo this, as the rest of the group may resent it.
  - If they are sensitive and nervous, compliment them sincerely the first time they make a contribution.
- *The rambler* talks about everything except the subject under discussion, and may use far-fetched analogies or lose the thread of what is happening. When such people stop for breath:
  - thank them and refocus their attention by summarising the relevant points
  - glance obtrusively at your watch.

- *If there is a personality clash.* This can factionalise your group and severely hamper discussion.
  - – Emphasise points of agreement.
  - – Draw attention back to the point of the meeting.
  - – Cut across the argument with direct questions on the topic.
  - – Restate group boundaries: 'we need to keep personalities and judgements out of the discussion'.
- *The obstinate group member.* Hasn't seen your point or perhaps is prejudiced and won't budge.
  - – Throw the view to the group and encourage him or her to comment briefly on it.
  - – Tell the person that time is short and that, while you will be glad to discuss it later, you would like him or her to accept the group's view for the moment.
- *The griper.* May have a legitimate complaint that is strongly felt, although this may be a pet peeve.
  - – Reiterate the objective of the discussion and the time pressures on the meeting.
  - – Point out the constraints under which everyone is operating.
  - – Suggest that they discuss the problem with you privately or raise the issue in a more appropriate forum.
- *Someone who has missed the point.* Take the blame and say: 'something I said must have led you off the subject. This is what we should be discussing ...'.
- *If group members are having a side conversation.*
  - – Do not order them to be quiet.
  - – Call them by name, restate the last opinion expressed by the group and ask their opinion of it.

If you are presenting a paper at a meeting:

- keep it brief, preferably one side of A4
- use bullet points to summarise text
- use coloured graphics or tables to illustrate concepts or massed information
- circulate copies for everyone to read before the meeting
- highlight individual responsibilities or action points for each participant.

Communication management

Managers should have strategies in place for clearly communicating the function and responsibilies within each job, and for managing the risk of staff failing to perform. Policies should be developed that observe current and future employment legislation and legal requirements.

Outward communication skills are becoming more important in general practice; managers also need to be PR and marketing experts. All employees are ambassadors for their organisation, and outward appearances count. The practice may have a mission statement where the partnership and staff values are spelt out. This, and any publicised standards displayed in the practice leaflet or charter, will be the image the public expects. It is important to work to these standards otherwise cynicism will set in; it is important the values are adhered to and shown to be working from the top.

Improve communication

Audit some of your operational systems to see if they are working at their best. For example, ensure that your telephone system, a key-operational system linking all internal and external communications, is best meeting the needs of your customers and staff.

Use the following methods to address any demonstrable communication difficulties. Aim to bring together staff and patients with an objective to seek common understandings and a shared vision of quality.

- Evaluate **qualitatively**, using a soft systems approach as a starting point.[4] Draw your present telephone system, noting any breakdowns in communication, with a focus on people's roles, conflicts and problems. Is there chaos and miscommunication or order and structure?
- Collate information and ideas from others – what are the issues of concern, what visions do they have, are these visions shared? Use the data to support your own observations.
- Construct a **quantitative** analysis using a patient questionnaire. Ask them how they experience the service, and what they would like to see change.
- Begin to think more widely around the issue:
  - What external pressures are shaping the organisation?
  - Who holds the power – patients, staff, doctors?
  - Where is the conflict and co-operation between the parties?
  - Who is dependent on whom?
  - Who has the power to sabotage?

The answers to these questions may help shape your recommendations. Established and previously understood relationships are changing in general practice; health service reforms have shifted the power base from doctors and their staff to the patients, who are resisting dependence. Patients are more confident about asking for what they want both in the type of service received and also the shape, or quality, of that service. Practices are having to develop new relationships with their customers.

There are other, more subtle, relationships to address. The balances of power between staff, and between the staff and their employers, the doctors – the influence of more invasive internal and external management presents a new and challenging dynamic. There is a new and developing relationship between the managers of healthcare and the clinicians – different roles, shifting attitudes and an emerging power base which is challenging to clinicians.

Look in further detail at your picture and compare this with a picture of your ideal. Where is communication breaking down? Where is customer focus lacking? Is your system all of the following.[5]

- Accessible?
- Equitable?
- Relevant to need – is there a discrepancy here between the practice and the patient's definition of need? Do patients expect general practice to be providing an emergency service for what the practice perceives as self-limiting illnesses?
- Efficient – do you deliver within available resources?
- Effective – is the service benefiting both client groups?

Make recommendations

How can your organisation make the changes required in order to meet the standards now required of it? This audit may well identify other quality issues that need addressing. Quality does cost but, as we have seen, the costs of not addressing it in a committed and systematic way are high. Practices who conduct audits in this way are already investing in a total quality management approach through attempting to **control** and monitor the process and to prevent problems through a systematic audit process (**quality assurance**). A **quality management** philosophy would require the commitment and involvement of everyone in the organisation.

Control and regulation in general practice is problematic, precisely because of the difficulty of making and maintaining agreement, as everyone tends to hold different judgements about acceptability. Hence the need to have an open debate, and then to develop agreed standardised procedures:

- Put in place some workable solutions to the current problem, e.g. who mans the telephone at peak times, having more direct lines, having a results only line.
- Audit other operational systems within the practice which involve patient services (e.g. repeat prescriptions, appointments) and remediate by recommending some robust, cost-effective and workable suggestions.

References

1   Wilson J (1995) General practice risk management. *News for Fundholders*. **4**.

2   Fred Pryor Seminars (1997) *How to Supervise People*. Pryor Resources Inc., Shawnee Mission, Kansas.

3   Martin V (2001) A meeting of minds. *Practice Manager*. **Dec/Jan**: 18–19.

4   Checkland P (1999) *Systems Thinking, Systems Practice*. Wiley, Chichester.

5   Maxwell R (1984) Quality assessment in health. *BMJ*. **288**: 1470–2.

Further reading

• Department of Health (1989) *Working for Patients*. CM555. HMSO, London.
• Department of Health (1991) *The Patients' Charter*. HMSO, London.
• Donabedian A (1980) The definition of quality: a conceptual exploration. In: A Donabedian (ed.) *Explorations in Quality Assessment and Monitoring*. Health Administration Press, Ann Arbor, Michigan.
• Hawksley N (2000) Paper chase. *Practice Manager*. **Aug**: 21–2.
• Øvretveit J (1992) *Health Service Quality: an introduction to quality methods for health services*. Blackwell Scientific, Oxford.
• Paton R *et al.* (1994) *Organisations: cases, issues, concepts*. Paul Chapman Publishing Ltd, London.
• Peter T and Waterman N (1985) *A Passion for Excellence*. Fontana/Collins, London.

Appendix A

An example induction pack

A planned induction gives general and detailed information on the practice. It should include:

- a formal letter of employment
- a contract
- an induction check list detailing:
  - practice facilities
  - procedures and protocols
  - staff names, main responsibilities and timetables
  - when and where the meetings are
  - who to contact if they need assistance
  - a list of local telephone numbers, e.g. hospital, pharmacy, social services.

Arrange for the new member of staff to be given:

- written information on how GPs are paid
- an introduction to the Red Book and IOS payments
- a pack of item of service forms with instructions on how to complete them.

They need to be made aware of:

- the current political position, e.g. the implications of The NHS Act 1999, PMS, the Clinical Governance Framework
- arrangements for private work and fees allowable
- the procedures for reimbursements
- any relevant clinical policies, e.g. prescribing formularies, NSF standards etc.

The practice manager can explain their role, and give further details about the financial and personnel management of a practice. An introduction to the management information (manual and computer systems) in use may be given as part of this induction.

Arrange for the inductee to spend time with:

- all the partners
- the accountant
- practice nurses
- senior receptionists
- attached staff.

Allow time for the employee to become familiar with the appointments and visits book, on call procedure, duty rota and telephone system. It is also very valuable for them to spend a morning in the waiting room, to experience what it is like for the patient attending the practice.

Appendix B

Letters and memos

When writing letters and memos:

- strive for clarity
- use the correct tone – formal or familiar
- correct paragraphing, spelling and punctuation
- format should follow organisational guidelines: introduction/reference, update or summary, possible action, polite closing. GPs can standardise their referral formats to include personal and drug history, presentation etc.
- give copies to everyone concerned.

Reports

Structure depends on whether the report is a personal account, routine or special report. Complex reports may require a detailed analysis of information or investigations, visual aids or action points.

Understand the purpose before researching and writing drafts. Structure with:

- a title and title page – with details of author, purpose of submission and submission date
- acknowledgements – to those who have assisted the author
- a table of contents – with sections and page numbers
- an introduction – the issue, problem, background, aim of investigation
- method used in the investigation
- content – background information, evidence, possible actions, costs and benefits
- summary – conclusion and recommendations
- references – identification of literature and sources used
- appendices – documents and bulky information which would clutter the text.

Appendix C

Telephone

The telephone is often the first point of call into general practice, so it is essential that it is answered in the correct manner. The caller will receive no visual clues, but can obtain a lot of information from the tone of voice. Whether a consultation call or an appointment request, consult and formally write a protocol, which covers the following points.

- All telephone calls must be answered within X rings; if you are busy with another patient, ask the caller to hold the line.
- Answer external calls with the name of the surgery followed by 'How can I help?'
- Answer internal calls with your name.
- Prioritise the emergency line.
- Identify yourself and name of business.
- Gather essential data – name, address and telephone number.
- Establish what the caller wants and why?
- Give administrative information if required.
- Examine the caller, verbally.
- Explore the options together.
- Make a decision.
- Take notes –avoid making callers repeat themselves.
- Ask for permission to place the caller on hold.
- If you are the caller, always call back if disconnected.

Voice mail

Leave clear, concise messages including:

- your name and organisation
- day and time
- purpose of call
- your telephone number.

For nurses

- Ensure protocols are in place for all delegated clinical procedures.
- Check registration status and training needs.

Visitors

- All patients and visitors to the practice are to be treated with equal courtesy and respect.
- Ask all visitors to sign in and out of the visitor's book, and give them a badge.
- When deliveries are signed in, telephone or leave a message with X member of staff.

Form filling

Correctly completed forms pay your wages.

- All forms must be completed in full to the set standard.
- Examples of all forms correctly filled are found in file X.
- Make sure the patient signs where indicated, and that all forms are dated correctly.
- Any wrongly completed forms will be retained in personal files for annual appraisal.

Messages

- Everyone must read the message book every day and names ticked once messages have been read.
- If leaving a message, sign your name.
- All written messages **must** contain:
  - your name
  - today's date.
- And, if applicable:
  - the full name and telephone number of the contact
  - the reason for calling.

Medical records

- The tracer system must always be used.
- Always double check if the patient has a same name sticker.

Conflict and complaints

- Remove the patient to a private space.
- Act promptly, and pass onto the appropriate person if the problem is not quickly solved.

Payments for non-GMS work

- Ensure the customer pays in full for any private medical services. Underpayment and IOUs are not acceptable.
- Inform the customer, when they make an appointment, that it is private work and that they may have to pay for some treatment, and ascertain which method of payment they would prefer.
- We accept cash and guaranteed cheques only.
- At the beginning and end of every day please ensure there is enough change in the petty cash tin.
- **Never** accept a cheque without a banker's card. Check the date, signature, and expiry date.
- Watch while the cardholder signs.
- Check the validity of dates.
- Check the cardholder's title, e.g. Mr/Mrs/Ms.
- If you are at all suspicious, you must obtain authorisation.

Ordering and stock control

- X is the only member of staff responsible for ordering all supplies, received in writing.
- Stock control is monitored monthly, and stock audits are held annually.

Appendix D

How effectively do you manage your meetings?

For each factor, circle a number that most represents your view of your own management of the meetings that you chair.

1 I spend the minimum amount of time in meetings and they are effective and well planned.   1 2 3 4 5   I spend far too much time in meetings and mainly they could be more effective.

2 I always plan ahead and clearly define the purpose of my meeting.   1 2 3 4 5   I rarely plan my meetings in advance and the purpose is probably unclear.

3 I always establish in my own mind that the meeting is cost-effective.   1 2 3 4 5   I very rarely attempt to establish whether my meetings are cost-effective.

4 I always try to keep my meetings to the minimum number of relevant people.   1 2 3 4 5   Probably my meetings have too many people and not all those people are necessarily relevant.

5 I spend time thinking carefully about my agenda and I always publish it in advance.   1 2 3 4 5   I rarely publish an agenda and, when I do, it is probably weak and sketchy.

6 Normally people are well prepared for my meetings.   1 2 3 4 5   I always have the common complaint that people are not well prepared for my meetings.

7 I always publish the finish time and allocate time properly to each agenda item.   1 2 3 4 5   I rarely publish a finish time and my time management could probably be improved fairly substantially.

8 I am very conscious of the need for good chairmanship and I actively try to improve my skills.   1 2 3 4 5   I am afraid that my chairmanship is haphazard.

9 At the end of each meeting   1 2 3 4 5   I often end a meeting
   I allocate time to summarising,   without ensuring that
   and ensure that all actions are   actions are clearly
   accountable.   accountable.

10 I always try to ensure that   1 2 3 4 5   Other people's meetings
    meetings where I am not   are their responsibility.
    chair are properly
    managed.

If you selected lower numbers, you have very firmly grasped that meetings need to be effectively managed and you are always conscious of the need to ensure good performance. Higher numbers need attention – your meetings will be low in effectiveness and not particularly productive for you or the participants. A consistent choice of number five means that you are wasting your time and everybody else's time in your meetings. Almost certainly the output of your meetings is very erratic.

CHAPTER 3

Understanding others

Personality

Good communicators understand and acknowledge personality differences and adapt their communication styles accordingly. What is it that makes people respond in particular, and sometimes maladaptive, ways? This chapter explores some of these personality traits, and encourages the reader to think more widely about their own personality and chosen ways of communicating.

Personality differences can either be a source of great strength and creativity or of conflict and, given that organisations consist of lots of people working together, managers need to be able to recognise this and harness the potential and talent available to meet the needs of the organisation. Leaders need to be able to understand what creates personality differences and be aware of the influences on their own attitudes and assumptions.

Organisations have their own personality. General practice is often run as a family business, with, in psychoanalytic terms, the people within behaving rather like a family, with the GPs behaving like the father or mother and staff within the practice finding their own family role.

Who, within your practice, acts out the roles of:

the father?

the mother?

the naughty child?

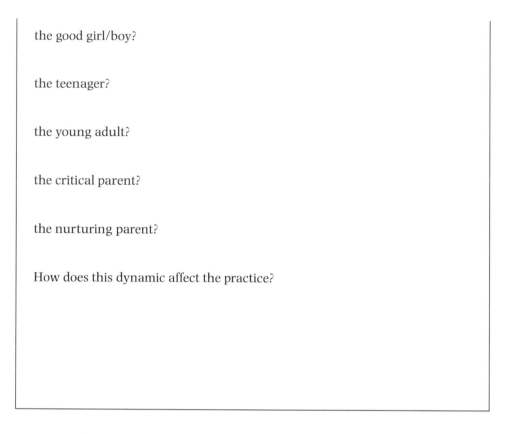

the good girl/boy?

the teenager?

the young adult?

the critical parent?

the nurturing parent?

How does this dynamic affect the practice?

Or try an idea from systemic family therapy – use pebbles to represent people, draw faces on them, place yourself in the centre and position the others as you feel they are in relation to you. Ask yourself, 'What is the current position?' 'Who supports whom?' Do the same exercise for yourself and your current family, your family of origin, and your position in the workplace. Are there any similarities?

Think how the people in your practice differ from each other in terms of:

- gender
- abilities
- physique
- values
- beliefs
- culture
- class
- communication styles
- what they want
- intellect.

People also demonstrate a whole range of talents, not all of which are commonly recognised and developed in the workplace. Amongst your colleagues you will find a range of musical, interpersonal, self-knowledge, spatial, sporting, scientific, artistic and creative abilities. Good leaders will recognise and develop all of these skills in those they manage.

We understand that **personality** is influenced by early developmental experiences (social, family and cultural) as well as adult experiences. Freud introduced us to the concept of defences; in childhood, we developed 'defences' that helped us deal with traumas, and these emerge later in adulthood when we are faced with difficult or stressful situations.[1] Managers have to hold this awareness – people will defend themselves when they do not want to be confronted with the difficult feelings again.

Some common defence mechanisms are:

- regression – adopting childish patterns of behaviour
- fixation – rigid and inflexible behaviour or attitudes
- rationalisation – 'covering up' of emotions with intellectual talk
- projection – attributing to others the feelings and motives we feel ourselves.

It is worth considering who in your practice demonstrates what personality traits. These can, of course be perceived as both strengths and weaknesses. Write down some of the personality traits of key people within your practice. Who is:

- practical
- serious
- casual
- logical
- dependable
- easy-going
- eager
- outspoken
- resourceful
- frank
- informed
- popular
- principled
- tolerant
- enthusiastic
- imaginative
- critical
- stubborn
- aggressive
- kind
- adaptable
- liberal
- considerate
- loyal
- unstable.

Motivation

A key part of any manager's task is maximising the staff's potential. Most of us could work harder with more commitment and interest, and produce higher quality work, with the right sort of encouragement. Motivation is simply the right encouragement for us. To perform well at work, people need:

- ability
- good working conditions
- motivation.

What is important for us to note is what it is that motivates people. Can we assume we know? Do you know what moves people to come to work, to achieve, to continue to persevere with difficulties? Think about key staff members. What do you really know about them, and what do you assume? Who:

- likes their work to be challenging
- likes to be popular with work mates
- always wants to lead the group
- likes to assume personal responsibility
- likes to set and achieve their own targets
- always shouts rather than talks
- seems to enjoy controlling other people
- becomes upset if forced to work on his/her own
- works very long hours
- tends to become bored when doing routine jobs
- tends to perform best when working in a team
- enjoys speaking to large groups
- carefully analyses and assesses problems.

In order to elicit the co-operation of staff and direct their performance to achieving the objectives of the organisation, managers must understand the nature of human behaviour. The difficulty is that the causes of behaviour are extremely complex and poorly understood. Often the cause of behaviour of the person we are observing is unknown to them although they might attempt to rationalise it. What chance does the manager have then?

What we do know about motivation is that:[2]

- employee behaviour is the result of forces in the individual and environment
- employees make conscious (and unconscious) decisions about their behaviour
- employees do what they see is rewarded, and avoid negative behaviour.

Theories of motivation

A person's motivation, job satisfaction and performance at work will be determined by both **extrinsic rewards**, such as salary and fringe benefits, and **intrinsic rewards**, the sense of challenge or achievement, positive recognition from the organisation, etc. People are influenced by the presence of:

- economic rewards (minor rewards are minor motivators)
- social relationships
- personal attitudes and values (seniority as the basis for promotion rewards the length of the employment, not the quality or quantity of performance)
- the nature of the work
- leadership styles
- satisfaction of the work itself.

Researchers such as Hertzberg[3] discovered which factors lead to extreme satisfaction.

- Achievement.
- Recognition.
- The work itself.
- Responsibility.
- Advancement.
- Growth.

And dissatisfaction.

- Policies and procedures.
- Relationship with supervisor and colleagues.
- Unsatisfactory working conditions.
- Salary/status.
- Job security.

Clearly, managers have to offer incentives appropriate to the individual's 'psychological' contract. In addition, they need to design jobs with:

- variety
- interest
- complexity
- challenge
- autonomy.

Maslow's basic proposition[4] was that people always want more, and what they want depends on what they already have. He demonstrated levels of need. If the lowest levels are met, the next level is sought. These levels are usually shown as a pyramid, with physiological needs at the bottom.

Maslow's Hierarchy of Needs:

- Self-actualisation (the development of one's full potential, challenge, creativity, achievement at work).
- Esteem needs (self-respect, achievement, status, recognition in the world).
- Love (social need to belong, affection, good professional associations and teamwork).
- Safety (freedom from threat or pain, the need for predictability and orderliness, job security, safe working conditions).
- Physiological (hunger, thirst, basic sensory satisfaction or – applied to work – satisfactory pay, good working conditions).

This hierarchy is not fixed, for some people other needs may compete. For one self-esteem may be more important than love; for the innately creative, the drive for self-actualisation may arise despite the lack of other needs met. Those who have been deprived of love in early childhood may experience the permanent loss of love needs or desire other forms of nourishment, like food. Someone who has never suffered chronic hunger may regard food as unimportant.

Individual differences mean that people place different values on the same need, and satisfaction is not necessarily the main motivational outcome of behaviour – job satisfaction does not necessarily lead to better work performance.

People need to be asked what motivates them at work. Most of us make judgements about human nature.

What do you assume?

- Most people are lazy and dislike work.
- For most people work is as natural as play or rest.
- People must be encouraged, or punished, if we are to achieve our organisational objectives.
- People like to exercise self-direction and control.
- People like to be committed to work.
- The average person avoids responsibility and prefers to be directed.
- We all like security.
- People accept responsibility readily.
- People work for money only.
- People work to achieve self-esteem and self-actualisation.

McGregor[5] argued that the following was more in line with reality.

- People are, by nature, motivated and it is only society and the working environment that frustrates their potential.

- People would like to contribute positively to the organisation of which they are members, if only they were given the opportunity.
- People will only follow leaders antagonistic to management when there are genuine, unrequited grievances or a lack of more positive leadership.

Do you understand your staff's motivational needs and are these taken into account when recruiting, or managing pay and reward systems?

The fact is people are different. Making assumptions about people creates misunderstandings and communication difficulties. If you understand and respect the differences in your workforce, they will be empowered, and there is more opportunity for you to encourage an increase in personal responsibility and initiative. You are giving individuals permission to be who they are, and this will help the development of better communication between you. People differ in the manner in which they satisfy needs. The following all affect responses.

- Cultural factors: affect the way in which we satisfy many of our leisure preferences.
- Perceptual factors: we see the world in terms of our own needs and as our needs change so does our view of our world.
- Abilities/aptitudes/personality.
- Frustration: one consequence of being unable to achieve a goal.
- Job satisfaction: relates to feelings about, and attitudes towards one's job.
- Absenteeism and turnover are related to job satisfaction but have little link with productivity.

Make a note on how your practice meets motivational needs. *See* Appendix A for some examples of how to improve motivation through improving communication. If the organisation does not meet people's motivational needs, they either adapt and seek an alternative goal, or become frustrated, and may show any of the following behaviours.[6]

Aggression	Physical or verbal attacks	Abusive language	
Destruction of equipment	Malicious gossip	Picking arguments	
Short-tempered	Sulking	Crying	Powerlessness
Temper tantrums	Fixed behaviour	Isolation	
Inability to accept change	Withdrawal	Resignation	Apathy
Sickness	Absenteeism	Avoidance	Alienation

How many of these are found in your organisation? Make a note here of some of the ways these behaviours can be reduced. Refer to Appendix A for some guidelines.

References

1   McLeod J (1998) *An Introduction to Counselling* (2e). Open University Press, Buckingham.

2   Fred Pryor Seminars (1997) *How to Supervise People*. Pryor Resources Inc., Shawnee Mission, Kansas.

3   Hertzberg F (1968) One more time: how do you motivate employees? *Harvard Business Review*. **46**: 53–62.

4   Maslow AH (1943) A theory of human motivation. *Psychological Review*. **50** (4): 370–96.

5   Adapted from McGregor D (1987) *The Human Side of Enterprise*. Penguin, Harmondsworth.

6   Mullins LJ (1999) *Management and Organisational Behaviour* (5e).   Financial Times Pitman, London.

7   Sourced from Brighton College of Technology course notes – *Supervision* (1997).

Appendix

How to improve staff motivation

- Develop a devolved management style, avoid top-heavy and authoritarian leadership.
- Encourage increases in personal responsibility and initiative.
- Develop more open dealings with staff, and avoid secrecy and manipulation.
- Discourage staff from seeking out and rewarding their favourite GPs – check to see which partners are favoured and why. (In some practices, it is only the men who get served with coffee and tea by the staff, for example.)
- Give staff opportunities for brief, frequent, informal gatherings to unwind and relax.
- Allocate regular coffee and tea breaks. Staff must be given protected time to socialise and relax.
- Increase salary benefits – people do not necessarily work better if they are highly paid, but they will work with less enthusiasm and commitment if they feel that they are paid below their current market rate. Make sure that people are paid according to their worth and value. Poor salary is the most usual reason for people to leave any organisation.
- Increase the opportunities for change and advancement – people need to feel they have a space to learn new skills or develop other aspects of their creative talent.
- Training. In order for people to perform their jobs effectively to your satisfaction and theirs, they will need training. Take the initiative to both supply and analyse training needs.
- Environment. Create physical comfort, and a relaxed 'feel' to the organisation.
- Counselling. If you wish to be in touch with your staff, be aware of their problems and what is affecting their work and performance – offer a counselling role.
- Information exchange. Keep people informed about what is happening in the organisation, what changes are occurring, and about new projects and new people. Provide them with the opportunity to let you know their thoughts and ideas about the organisation.
- Performance review. People need to be told clearly and understandably how they are performing and their strengths and weaknesses should be pointed out. This stops problems from developing and keeps you in touch. At the same time it gives them an opportunity to reflect upon how your management of them is helping or hindering their performance.
- Job descriptions. These are the tool by which the manager can ensure that the staff member has a clear and precise knowledge of the job,

its responsibilities, and its limits – a lack of which is a major source of grievance for employees. Define the nature of the job, its objectives and functions and then set it out in sensible priority order.

- Select the correct motivational stimulus in order to reduce the need for continual direction.
- The best motivator is the formation of cohesive, well-integrated groups.
- Satisfactory hygiene or 'maintenance' factors are the minimum for 'base' performance – wages, security, hours of work, general work environment.
- For superior performance consider group motivation, loyalty, power, companionship, status of person and group.
- Note the importance of providing for, and recognising, achievement.
- Job enrichment – add vertically to job to provide greater interest and opportunity for achievement. Allow worker to plan, and set targets and performance standards. Reduce supervision.

Ineffective techniques[7]

- Competition. The race for supremacy is counter-productive.
- Job rotation. It doesn't help to move from one boring job to another.
- Horizontal loading or job enlargement. More work is not satisfactory – it must be more interesting work.
- Reducing supervision does not mean greater responsibility. The employee may feel neglected.

CHAPTER 4

Teams, groups and facilitation

In this chapter we look at:

- what groups and teams are
- why team working is important
- how to build successful teams and groups.

Team working

A **team** is a **group** of people working together to achieve common goals. Team working can help:

- improve communication
- learning
- develop a sense of belonging
- build co-operation
- develop mutual support
- motivate staff
- achieve more.

The advantages are that:

- each person on a team has the chance to contribute their unique knowledge and be recognised for their contributions
- individuals achieve more working in teams than they could alone
- management can ensure everyone agrees on the objectives and nature of the working relationship.

The way clinicians, managers and inter-related services are working together with specific and shared responsibilities for healthcare provision is a new approach for the NHS. The Government vision of healthcare delivery is centred on teamwork. We have:

- more integrated/seamless care

- multidisciplinary team working
- disappearing boundaries between primary, secondary, and social care.

For this way of working to be successful, a representative from each professional group has to meet regularly to define and agree the boundaries and the ways in which they wish to work. This method of working is espoused in the Total Quality Management literature. Integrated and effective working visions are shared and involvement and co-operation are obtained from everyone. Team working needs emotional and practical investment from everyone in the organisation, especially the leaders. It is easier if:

- the business culture is relaxed and accommodating, not fixed and bureaucratic
- communication is good
- staff are kept informed
- their concerns are acted upon and not ignored
- everyone's views are respected.

Team working is not easy. The team needs to find a balance between the needs of the:

- task – do the task objectives fit with organisational objectives?
- team – what are the group objectives as a whole?
- individual – who will want to contribute, challenge, and may need authority to carry out delegated tasks.

What do you think makes teams effective?

Effective teams:

- recognise and value different roles of members
- are highly structured, problem focused and goal orientated
- keep clear records
- share ownership and common purpose
- set clear goals for each contribution from each discipline
- encourage participation
- communicate openly internally and externally
- support innovation and offer opportunities for learning and development
- confront conflict

- give feedback to each other
- have external recognition
- have diverse skills and personalities
- problem solve
- regularly review and process how they are working
- agree on common goals
- share a commitment to quality
- keep the same standards
- meet regularly
- promote ideas sharing
- listen actively to each other
- provide constructive criticism
- appreciate each other's skills
- respect diversity
- build trust
- are accountable for their own performance, as well as that of other team members
- are no more than 25 in number.

Teams have their own growth process.

- Exploring.
- Experimenting.
- Co-operating.
- Performing.

Teams progress through various stages of development. Rarely is this progression made in a linear or consistent fashion. As teams struggle to cope with rapidly changing internal or external events or variations in team membership they will progress or regress through the levels. Progress is most assured when teams consciously acknowledge or address the need to develop or tackle the reforming issues raised by change. Teams that do not take this into account are likely to regress to earlier stages of development despite the length of time that they have been working together, and this inevitably affects their performance.

Four stages of team development:[1]

Tentative/exploring: the tentative team is newly formed, with a great deal of uncertainty and lack of clarity.

Experimenting: this team tries out many ways of operating and relating, with a great deal of conflict, anger and unfocused energy.

Amalgamating/co-operating: here the team begins to forge strong working relationships, and starts to focus more readily on achieving results, whilst minimising destructive patterns of behaviour.

Maturing/performing: the maturing team has learned to operate effectively, whilst still recognising the need to continue to attend to team dynamics.

Eight ways to make a team fail.

- Don't give them a base or leader.
- Keep objectives and decision-making procedures vague.
- Never review the team's performance.
- Ignore the wider organisation.
- Have a high proportion of part-time team members.
- Encourage professionals to recruit, allocate work etc. to their own profession.
- Insist each professional group have their own referral procedures.
- Keep each profession meeting separately just as before the team began.

Groups

Groups are people who share the same task. Each person working within the group will have their own:

- personal and professional loyalties
- desires for status and power
- emotions, fears and anxieties
- skills, knowledge base, and authority.

This combination can be heady, and the group will do their utmost to find common ground to enable them to work together comfortably. As the group forms, it will unconsciously start to develop shared patterns of perceiving, thinking and communicating to counteract these feelings of individual isolation. Group members converge towards 'norms', and anyone who does not conform to those norms will be under pressure by the group to do so.

These norms may be:

- overt: task orientated, time/date of meeting, procedures
- covert: attitudes, dress codes, appearance, who sits next to who.

Devolve to involve

A more modern, inclusive way of working is to use teams and groups for all decision-making. One or two key people should not make decisions unilaterally. If this method is adopted, a culture develops so that:

- staff feel respected and empowered
- the culture shifts from one where people are passive and dependent and resentful of change, to one where they are more confident and innovative
- organisation is clearer, roles and responsibilities are centrally understood and defined
- there is more control and potential for growth
- results happen and decisions are made collectively, not autocratically or through independent management action

- better communication occurs, everyone begins to understand each other's working patterns and recognises others' stresses
- harmonisation of working practice occurs.

This kind of culture adapts well to change. Because the change operates from within and is not top led, it is cultivated rather than managed; there is an attitude of growth and learning, not instruction or control. The organisation moves towards a people-centred approach, where people, not tasks, become the focus of management.

Achieving groups:

- co-operative
- are active
- advance
- have a mission
- demonstrate leadership
- demonstrate environment responsiveness.

Co-operate
- Positively.
- Share information and feelings.
- Listen.
- Collaborate.
- Confront constructively.
- Support.
- Work to maintain excellent interpersonal relationships.

Are active
- Use systematic but adaptable work practices.
- Make decisions.
- Consider alternatives.
- Delegate.
- Ensure that the team achieves the brief.
- Individuals are clear about their own and other roles and competencies.
- Use different team roles to contribute to the aims of the team.
- Balance individual strengths while acknowledging and coping with limitations.

Advance
- Reviews its experiences.
- Individuals alter behaviour to enhance individual and group performance.
- Actively develops capacity to meet new challenges and demands.

Have a mission
- A shared and clear view of their goals.
- Adopt an action orientated approach towards their achievement.

Demonstrate leadership
- Stimulate high performance.
- Is responsive to the task.
- Support and reward team members.
- Can reside in one person or be shared and operate flexibly.

Demonstrate environment responsiveness
The team scans and responds to the environment to identify trends, ideas and opportunities and actively promote its mission.

Working in groups

- Ensure groups are aware of some of the 'softer' management issues: group dynamics, time management.
- Never stop sharing what you have learnt.
- Involve the main stakeholders – the GPs – put them right in the middle of the planning team. Use this energy, enthusiasm and lead to give everyone permission to change.

To be successful, groups must:

- have autonomy
- have accountability
- have authority
- have responsibility
- have a budget
- meet regularly
- have a self-defined remit, formed and owned through discussion with individual group members
- be formally defined, with a quorum, agendas and written minutes.

Key principles

- Group participants may consult outside of the group.
- Keep the emphasis on achievement, positive results, decisions made and problems solved.
- Each group sets their own objectives and targets.
- Outsiders must avoid interfering in decisions and actions made by the groups. It is important for the group to see their own ideas and initiatives taking shape.

Through using this approach, meetings become much shorter and more constructive – changes and ideas are presented, actioned, and outcome-based.

Group dynamics

Researchers have shown that groups go through certain processes in their development. Tuckman noted that groups pass through different stages in their development.[2] The stages are not linear – a group may regress back to an earlier stage under pressure or stress.

This is a natural phenomenon of groups and the wise leader/manager will acknowledge this and not try to prevent it happening but rather will allow the group space to experience the earlier stage and then, when the time is ripe, gradually bring the group back to the present task.

Five stages of group development:

Dependency: members may:

- feel dependent on the group leader
- feel resentful, confused and anxious
- expect to be told what to do
- be defensive and not take any risks
- question the leader a lot.

Conflict: the group may begin to:

- feel more confident
- set their own agendas
- challenge the leader
- form internal competition for leadership position
- see the emergence of an informal leader and subgroups
- criticise each other, hidden agendas may emerge.

Togetherness: members begin to feel

- good about being a member of the group
- 'we' feelings, feelings of togetherness
- that the group has become a rewarding experience for the members
- more openness, sharing information relevant to the task
- a productive phase of group life.

Beware of the group becoming stuck in the 'feel good' mode and not address-ing the task. Communication patterns may become rigid.

Interdependence:

- often not reached by many groups
- groups perform optimally with good interpersonal relationships evident
- task-focused
- members feel able to criticise each other without it being taken personally
- commitment to the team is high
- goals and purpose of the team is 'owned' by the members
- flexibility of working practices exist towards individual, subgroups or the whole team
- highly creative phase of working together.

Loss/grieving: members may feel:

- threatened by the ending of the group or by the prospect that the group will achieve its task and cease to exist
- sad, and attempt to resist the ending of the group.

Facilitating groups

Good facilitators learn their skill. The group facilitator needs to be able to encourage differing viewpoints while supporting the discussion, keep time and ensure everyone present sticks to the subject.

The role of the facilitator is to:

- extract feelings and ideas from the audience
- summarise the content of the meeting
- help pull the ideas of a group together
- enable the group to move forward
- help the group achieve a successful outcome.

A good facilitator will:

- welcome a group
- co-ordinate their activities
- keep charge of events
- follow and accompany the group rather than lead it
- intervene where necessary
- achieve successful outcomes.

Belbin[3] noted different personality types are found within groups, and each needs to be skilfully managed (*see* Table 4.2).

How do you perform in a group? Can you:

- work well with a wide range of people
- draw people out
- produce ideas

Table 4.1

Task	Activity	Features
Forming dependence	Define the nature and boundaries of task	Group members concerned with why they are there Interpersonal relationships and boundaries are tested Dependency on leader develops Uncertainty and anxiety are felt Commitment to group is low Grumbling about task Behaviour meandering and ineffective Suspicion of task and each other Testing and confronting behaviour Hesitating or avoiding task
Storming	Questioning the value of exercise	Conflict occurs Members resist task and group influences Arguments about what the purpose of the group is Members may undermine each other and the leader Authority is questioned People jockey for position within the group Challenging behaviour Experimenting with hostility, aggression, frustration, rivalry, resentment, opposition Defensive behaviour
Norming	Opening up and inviting	New roles adopted by group members Resistance to group overcome Expressions of intimate, personal opinions around the goal Feelings of belonging to the group and identification with the group as a unit emerge Commitment goes up Defining tasks Evaluating Mutually supportive Showing unity and consensus Liking each other
Performing/ interdependence	Effectively pursuing the task	Group energy directed towards completion of task Creative problem solving Roles become flexible and functional Frequent and mutual contributions Interpersonal issues now disregarded or sorted or used as a tool to achieve goals of groups Feel safe and confident Achieving
Ending/ mourning	Facing the loss of the group experience	Denial of ending Termination phase Group dissolves because task is completed Group resists disintegration through social contact Fantasising about the 'good old days' may begin, idealising the past history of the group This may occur when interpersonal issues prevent the group from accomplishing its task Bargaining, anger or depression may occur Group may perform rituals

Table 4.2

Personality type	Plus points	Potential difficulties
Completer/finisher	Likes detail Will complete a task Can concentrate Good judgement skills Meets deadlines High standards Very accurate	Can be pedantic Poor tolerance of 'casual' or flippant behaviour Can be over-anxious or introvert
Implementer	Practical Systematic Disciplined Loyal Reliable Efficient	Can be rigid

Monitor/evaluator	Able to analyse problems,
	  ideas and options
	Good judgement skills
		Serious minded and cautious,
		  could upset the casual worker
		Slow thinker
		Can be critical

Specialist	High professional
	  standards
	Expert in narrow field
	In-depth knowledge
	  and experience
		Not broad minded
		Lacks interest in other subjects

Team worker	Mild
	Sociable
	Supportive and concerned
	  about others
	Diplomatic, flexible,
	  adaptable
	Sensitive, perceptive to
	  needs of team
	Good listener
	Popular
	Good at raising morale,
	  reducing conflict and
	  promoting co-operation
		Can be indecisive

Resource
  investigator
	Enthusiastic
	Extrovert
	Relaxed
	Inquisitive
	Good communicator
	  and negotiator
	Can think on their feet
	Develops other's ideas
	Investigates contacts
	  and resources
		Needs constant stimulation
		  of others

Table 4.2   Continued

Personality type	Plus points	Potential difficulties
Shaper	Single-minded, extrovert, strong drive	Competitive, aggressive, challenging
	Thrives under pressure	Pushy
	Achiever	Can be frustrated
	Good at overcoming obstacles	May lack understanding of others
	Prepared to take unpopular decisions	
Plant	Creative innovator	Unorthodox
	Good at generating new ideas	Impractical
		Poor communicator
	Can solve complex problems	Sensitive to praise or criticism

Note how people behave in your group.

Discuss these behaviours with the group and ask them to seek out ways of reinforcing positive behaviour and challenging negative behaviour. Be aware of who:

- takes initiative
- takes leadership
- offers directions
- seeks suggestions
- encourages others
- makes helpful suggestions
- tries to solve problems
- calms things down
- encourages compromises
- acts as spokesperson
- chairs
- notes down the minutes
- is obstructive or negative
- checks progress
- keeps time
- builds on ideas
- challenges appropriately
- generates ideas
- criticises
- offers irrelevant ideas.

- face temporary unpopularity if it leads to worthwhile gains in the end
- retain a steadiness of purpose in spite of the pressures
- influence people without pressurising them

- foster good working relationships
- lead from the front.

Or do you:

- lose track and get caught up in the ideas
- talk too much
- feel reluctant to join in
- retire when the going gets tough
- get irritated when no progress is made
- hesitate to get your point across
- demand things of others when not prepared to do them yourself
- show impatience with those obstructing progress.

Some people have difficulty containing the confidences shared within the group. There is a need for boundaries and confidentiality within the group. Where do you see yourself in this list of containers? Which one would people most confide in?

The chipped, leaky jar	–	A risky choice.
The plastic medicinal model	–	Holds exactly the right number of contents and has a child proof cap.
The rose vase	–	Rather narrow, difficulty getting things in or out.
The wide necked vase	–	Transparent. Easier filling, and fairly flexible, but no lid available so contents might fall out.
The casserole pot	–	Plenty of space, firm, good lid for keeping contents secure when required.
The jam jar	–	Contains other things already.
The locked tin box	–	Far too rigid. Extremely difficult to get into. Contents not visible.
The pillbox	–	Very small container, secure, useful for treasures.
Small, soft leather duffle	–	Flexible, but limp and rather unsafe.

Facililitators:

- discover individual needs and try to get those needs met
- address and balance conflict
- give priority to doubts and uncertainties
- tolerate criticism.

Facilitation means:

Preparing – Managing – Summarising.

- Keeping to the agenda.
- Keeping to time.

- Allowing useful debate.
- Involving everyone.
- Encouraging creativity.
- Making decisions.
- Agreeing on actions.

The ideal facilitator has certain features. *See* the Appendix for these and mark off those you can see in yourself.

Managing difficulties in groups

Here are some common problems for groups:

Not enough time   Group badly managed   Apathetic
People abuse confidentiality   Too many interruptions   Dr B opts out
Unenthusiastic   Group stuck   Names and titles not negotiated
Staff member hogs the time
Members not clear about the purpose of meeting
C ignores non-verbal cues   F tries to be leader   Unsuitable room
Red herrings brought up endlessly
Subgroups forming   Boundaries not defined
Dr P's hidden agenda   Meets erratically   M point scoring
Inappropriate teasing and harassment
Anti-authority   Does not respect rules of confidentiality

We have already looked at some ways we can best manage groups. We know the following can help.

- Be alert – notice all that happens in the group.
- Be aware that group dynamics can be very powerful so facilitators may experience strong emotions as well as the group.

Everyone within the group will have their own defence mechanisms, which may make people appear rigid and inflexible. These mechanisms are important in keeping people comfortable and within their 'safe zone'. If what you have to say challenges, do not set out to destroy these defences but challenge gently in different, less confronting, ways: 'It sounds as though you have strong feelings about that – I wonder what it is that has led you to feel that way.'

- Keep your language reflective, open and non-judgemental.
- Be provocative and challenging, yet gently curious.

- Be aware of your own prejudices/feelings and behaviour.
- Stand back – separate the process from the content.
- Intervene at group rather than individual level: 'the group seems too full of tension and unspoken anger'.

You do not have to understand everything that occurs in a group immediately – any significant or difficult behaviour will undoubtedly recur. You can manage difficult groups by:

- splitting them up, or changing the room set-up
- setting a task enabling the issues to be addressed
- using wide gestures and voice control – or silence
- using a flip chart
- have a break or early lunch, then change the set-up of the room.

Manage difficult individuals by:

- asking them to summarise so far
- inviting them to contribute to the whole group by talking about it or using a flip chart
- asking them to scribe
- using individual names as a controlling mechanism
- inviting the difficult individual to contribute to the whole group – or get them on your side
- using the skills of other team members
- at a pinch, take difficult members outside and discuss their behaviour with them.

Anticipate problems in advance.

- There may be a need for group mentoring: who can assist if a group is not functioning well?
- Check the number of groups within an organisation: there is never enough time for yet more meetings. Identify the essential ones, then dissolve or amalgamate others.
- Value meetings and any outcomes.
- Plan meetings in work time so staff are paid to attend, or fund catering needs.
- Give groups a clear leader, remembering someone will emerge anyway if unelected.
- Keep groups as small as possible. In a group of eight people, there are eight different agendas but potentially 28 different relationships going on.

Teach groups how to best function.[4] Forewarn them:

- about group dynamics (personality types to be found within groups and how to manage them)

- about non-verbal behaviour
- of the tendency for men to interrupt women or dominate the space
- that oppression rules: the 'experts' and higher social class will dominate
- to be sensitive to quieter members and give them space
- how groups develop
- of some 'best practice' ideas around meetings management, e.g. be prompt, no side talking, keep to time.

If the group has problems:

- *Your group has a compulsive talker.* Agree to divide the time for a short period and take turns in speaking so that everyone has a chance to give an opinion.
- *People are reluctant to talk.* Divide into pairs. It's often easier to talk to one person rather than several. Share your ideas and then report back to the rest of the group.
- *You spend most of your time just 'chatting'.* Perhaps members do not know where to start or are unprepared. Think about and discuss an overall agenda.
- *The group feels unsettled.* People can be made to feel anxious about giving opinions and talking openly if the group becomes overtly critical and judgemental. Create a supportive and open environment where all opinions can be heard, without making people feel insecure or unsupported.
- *Issues of vital academic importance arise.* Agree that you need some more help. Find a colleague who may be able to help.
- *Group members are 'freeloading'.* Return to your group agreement and re-negotiate your group's rationale. However, the benefits of explaining and working are much greater than simply listening so 'workers' will gain much more than 'freeloaders'; you should not give up if you feel some people are contributing more than others.

Guidelines for small group discussion:

- Speak in the first person: 'I think ...' 'I feel ...' (instead of you, we or one!).
- Avoid judgements: 'That's stupid ...' 'You shouldn't do that.'
- Avoid sarcasm or taking over what someone else is trying to practice for him/herself.
- Beware of giving advice which stems from your own experience. Although it may be correct, it is important to remember that there are no right answers, only a number of alternatives.
- Practice giving helpful, positive feedback as well as helpful critical feedback. This applies particularly to body language which the person may well be unaware of. They can use the feedback to improve their management of the situation.
- Do not overwhelm the person practising with remarks and suggestions during role-play. Wait until there is a pause.

Good facilitators:

- understand group dynamics
- have excellent interpersonal skills
- have good chairing skills
- are able to team build
- can manage conflict
- have good first line counselling skills
- do not 'perform'.

The communication skills required are to:

- welcome
- co-ordinate
- manage
- control
- discern
- listen
- watch
- summarise.

Facilitate change by:

- being open
- encouraging trust
- approving/validating
- allowing tension release through acknowledging emotions
- eliciting information
- inhibiting irrelevant conversation and side-talk
- understanding group process
- reflecting back to the group
- contributing
- handing over and/or taking control as needed.

References

1   Cook A (1997) *How Capable is Your Team?* Salomans Centre, Kent.

2   Tuckman BW (1965) Development sequences in small groups. *Psychological Bulletin.* **63**: 384–99.

3   Belbin RM (1991) *Management Teams: why they succeed or fail.* Heinemann, London.

4   Middleton J (2000) *The Team Guide to Communication.* Radcliffe Medical Press, Oxford.

Further reading

- Adair J (1993) *Effective Teambuilding*. Pan, London.
- Hunt J (1992) *Managing People at Work: A manager's guide to behaviour in organisations* (3e). McGraw-Hill, London.
- Janis IL (1968) *Victims of Group Think: a psychological study of forming policy decisions and fiascos*. Houghton Mifflin, Boston.
- Martin V (2001) A meeting of minds. *Practice Manager*. **Dec/Jan**: 18–19.

Appendix

The ideal facilitator:

- knows their subject, has credibility and presence but is not arrogant
- has broad shoulders and good interpersonal skills
- is self-aware
- is self-assured and assertive but not bossy and insensitive
- has common sense but does not enforce their views
- is a good organiser
- is particular about detail without being rigid
- is non-judgmental and neutral
- has the ability to listen and has awareness of group dynamics
- is a clear leader without being bossy
- is resilient and confident
- is sympathetic and diplomatic
- can motivate, energise and stimulate
- is articulate, direct and clear
- can conceptualise and think flexibly
- is patient
- has the ability to stand back and separate process from content
- gets on well with all people
- is a fast learner
- does not overrun
- never hits group members!

CHAPTER 5

Communicating in organisations

We have looked at communication between individuals and groups; now we take a broader look at communication in the context of larger groups, or organisations. Nothing happens in any organisation without people. But the study of organisations involves more than just the behaviour of people, and this needs to be put into context. To fully understand your organisation's communication processes, you need to have a broad understanding of:

- management processes
- the organisational context, processes and interactions
- people, and why they behave as they do.

You will now have an idea of some of the management processes in your organisation, and some idea of the motivations and goals sought by those within your organisation. However, people do not work in isolation. What impacts on your organisation, and what influences behaviour within it?

- The individual?
- The (formal or informal) group they belong to?
- The organisation?
- The environment?

Many things influence the NHS.

- Patients.
- Technology.
- The Government.
- Facilities.
- Rules and regulations.
- Financial constraints.
- Scientific development.

Structure is created by management to create order, to help establish relationships between people, and to direct the efforts of the organisation towards the goals they have established. Behaviour is affected by these systems.

More covert behavioural aspects also influence organisations.

- Attitudes.
- Communication.
- Team processes.
- Personalities.
- Conflict.
- Political behaviour.
- Underlying competencies and skills.

It is the role of the manager to understand and integrate all these activities, to co-ordinate, encourage and improve systems and people, and to ensure that people's work needs are satisfied.

Most of us are unaware of just how much culture affects us. General practice is influenced not just by the pervading external cultural factors (language, values, religion, education, the law, economics, politics, technology, environment, attitudes),[1] but also by its own internal culture. The internal culture could be heavily influenced by the history of the development of medicine, where the values may be old-fashioned, patriarchal and conservative, or set by others with different views and values.

- What are the influences in your practice? Religion, family, conservatism?
- How far do your own values coincide with the practice values?
- Do you fit in, or are you lost?

These values affect the ways in which people will accept, and tolerate, leadership. As flexible, short term working patterns become more common, people are less likely to feel a need to conform to the work values. The social and 'family' function of work is becoming less important. For GPs the picture changes depending on whether they are salaried or contracted. One brings more freedom, the other more commitment. As working practices become more informal, managers may need to work harder to support their practices to work together to achieve common core values.

The organisational context

Organisations come in all shapes and sizes, but there are common factors. There are always two broad categories of resources.

- Non-human – physical assets, materials, equipment, facilities.
- Human – people's abilities and skills, and their influence.

In all organisations, whatever their size, we see the **efforts** and interactions of people working to **achieve objectives** through a **structure** which is directed and **controlled** by management.

Formally, organisations operate with organisational charts, policies and procedures; informally, through personal friendships, grapevines, emotions, power games, and informal relationships and leadership.

Traditionally, organisations can be distinguished in terms of two generic groups, private enterprise or public sector. General practice currently, and sometimes uncomfortably, straddles the two. While the 'red book' contract still stands, there will always be an inherent tension between the care-taking quality and the need to make money.

Think about the key characteristics within your organisation.[2]

- Size   –   Small or very large?
- Formality   –   Informal or highly structured?
- Activities   –   What tasks are performed? By whom?
- Complexity   –   Simple or complicated?
- People skills   –   Types of people involved – class, education, age, etc.
- Location   –   Single or multiple?
- Goals   –   What is the organisation trying to accomplish?

Stakeholders

Stakeholders are people who have an interest and/or are affected by the goals or activities of the organisation.

Identify your stakeholders.

- Employees
- The health authority
- PCG/T
- The providers of finance – public and private
- Consumers – customers and patients
- Community and environment
- Government

- What do they want from you?
- How do they exert their power and influence?
- How do you communicate with them?

Who do you see as your business partners? Are their ideas welcomed?

Think about who drives the cultural change, and who resists the change. One of our management roles is to successfully manage change, to ensure we move beyond the status quo by either reducing the impact of some of the driving forces (enabling the resisters to move forward), or influence those resisting so that they come to realise the need for change themselves. One of the biggest learning points in doing this exercise is to see how far we push change, without enabling people to take it on board themselves.

Ask yourself:

- who drives the change in your organisation?
- who has the biggest influence?
- why do we resist change?

We need to be aware of these barriers, in ourselves and in those we manage.

If your practice has a person-centred culture,[3] with a powerful and autocratic style of leadership and management attempting to manage, there will be an equally powerful force within the practice resisting this type of management. There will be others within the practice that make formal or informal bids for leadership at different times, which complicates matters even further!

Your practice may work as a 'galaxy of stars' with each GP making a bid for leadership at different times. It is never clear, within this type of practice, who leads, and chaotic management results. There will also always be powerful internal and external forces pushing all practices into change, which is viewed by some in the organisation as positive, and by others as negative.

If these cultural forces are recognised and understood, they can be worked with, and both the practice and those within it would benefit through a reduction in stress and conflict.

It is clear that many practices are not managed successfully and sensitively. There are too many time pressures which lead both the managers and partners to manage badly in an autocratic, chaotic or uninformed way, even if their preferred style might be more enabling. There is too little understanding of management and organisation to enable managers to manage successfully.

Each practice has to review how their organisation works, and their management role. This means involving the whole team, looking at those tasks that can be taken on by other leaders in the organisation (the office manager, the accountant, the partners). Whatever decisions are made, it is imperative that the whole organisation is involved at whatever level, and for everyone to be clear about those decisions.

There is not necessarily ever a best or right way to do things – this depends on the task and the state of the organisation at the time. Whatever option is chosen there needs to be awareness and flexibility around managing both the process and the outcome.

Culture and leadership

Leadership styles can give us a clue as to the type of culture within your organisation. Managers all have their own individual way of leading. In general practice, the culture is usually hierarchical, with the staff responsible to the manager, but accountable to the partners who own the business. If the management and partnership styles differ difficulties can arise. The power base shifts, staff bypass the manager to clarify issues and management credibility and authority is lost. This weakens the organisation and can set up uncertainties and confusions as management is undermined.

There are several ways to manage, most managers adopt a style that they feel comfortable with and match the expectations of the people they work for. Each style carries its own strengths and weaknesses, and the reader will recognise their own approach.

Can you recognise the leadership style in your practice? Below are some examples of each style.

Autocratic management

The people who respond best to this style are those who need clear, detailed and achievable directives.

- This is safe and paternalistic.
- It carries a clear chain of command and authority.
- The divisions of work and hierarchy are fully understood by all.
- It works well in a crisis, or in a situation where quick results are needed.

The weaknesses are in the apparent efficiency of one-way communication – as we know, without feedback there is often misunderstanding and communication breakdown. The critical weakness, however, is its effect on people – most people resent authoritarian rule and respond with resentment, resistance or sabotage. The authoritarian ruler does not respect people and this causes low morale.

Bureaucratic management

People feel secure with this type of leadership.

- There is a consistency of policy and operations.
- There is a sense of fairness and impartiality.
- People know and understand the rules.

Although directives, policies and rules are essential in any business, there must be some flexibility, otherwise people react as they would to autocratic management. It is important to be flexible in situations where there should be exceptions to rules, to remember that polices represent legislation for the majority. Paralysis can result if the rules are ambiguous. Although it is tidier where approaches are uniform, procedures regular and there is accountability for operations, this can lead to unquestioning adherence to specified rules and procedures. This can be limiting and stifles flexibility, creativity and freedom. Of course, tried and tested rules and procedures help to ensure essential values and ethics, and this helps to ensure consistency and fairness.

Does your practice work in this way? What do you see as the advantages and disadvantages of this approach?

- Clear cut hierarchies and procedures.
- High levels of specialisation can be achieved.
- Uniformity of decisions and actions.
- A clear structure of authority.
- Good co-ordination.
- Rational, impersonal judgements are made.
- Life long career expectations.
- Dependence on rules and regulations.

Diplomatic management

- Commonly seen in general practice.
- Manager has no real line of authority.
- Manager dependent on the skills of persuasion in getting the co-operation needed.

Here the manager takes time to explain rather than order – this has advantages in that people work more enthusiastically if given reasons for a task and they feel respected. The manager is rewarded by co-operation. Often staff recognise the attempts to persuade rather than order as a sign of weakness, and can lose respect for the manager. If the diplomacy fails, the manager fails to 'sell' the deal, this comes through to people as frank manipulation and hypocrisy, and is thus deeply resented and resisted. The manager has lost out by not having a clear-cut line of authority – any attempt then to revert to a frank autocratic order has an obvious and disastrous effect on people.

Free-rein management

- Delegation optimises full use of time and resources.
- Many people are motivated to full effort if given freedom.

This carries a high degree of risk with very little managerial control – the manager needs to know the competence and integrity of the staff and their ability to handle this kind of freedom. It is a level of management usually given only to senior managers in an organisation.

Participative management

Each leadership style has its own pros and cons, but the benefits of participation outweigh the cons.

- Encourages wide communication.
- The manager benefits from a rich array of good information and ideas.
- Improves decision-making.
- Averts disaster.
- People are encouraged to develop.
- People contribute more.
- People develop a sense of personal achievement and value.
- People work better and more enthusiastically when given a high level of freedom in contribution.
- The work climate unleashes power, gives people recognition and a deep sense of personal value and esteem.
- People support decisions instead of fighting them.
- They work hard to make it work, because it becomes their idea.

The down side.

- It takes time.
- It can be inefficient if used inappropriately.
- Some people are not bright or committed enough to take on board the responsibility it releases.
- Managers may use this style as a way of devolving or abdicating responsibility.
- If not handled well, it can result in a complete loss of managerial control.

Are you:

- **Autocratic**: the manager tells not sells.
- **Bureaucratic**: the manager abides by the rules and regulations.
- **Diplomatic**: the manager takes time to explain rather than order.

- **Free-rein management**: over-delegation carries a high degree of risk with little managerial control.
- **Participative management**: staff have a key input into decision-making.

Use the following examples to think again how different people are in their values, approaches and personalities. Appreciate how difficult it is to adopt one leadership style that everyone would value.

- I value stability in my job.
- I like my life to be unpredictable.
- If I could afford it, I would prefer to be self-employed or freelance.
- Rules and procedures tend to frustrate me.
- I like working flexibly.
- I like uniforms.
- I feel constrained by organisations that are too tidy and predictable.
- Rules are meant to be broken.

Think about these key influences on the culture of general practice.

- History – when and why did the NHS form? What was the background to general practice development? How are GPs seen in relation to their consultant colleagues?
- What do you see as the primary function of general practice? What is the importance of reputation? The range of services provided?
- What are the prime goals and objectives? Money? Patient care? Excellence?
- Size and location: What are the communication difficulties presenting? What about opportunities for development?
- Management influences: Are you responsive to change? Is anyone else in the practice?
- What are the routines, rituals and stories told within the organisation, and within the NHS as a whole?
- What symbols are used by the practice – any logos, titles, language used that represent the practice to outsiders?

Organisational structure

Here we look at the basic framework within which the manager's decision-making behaviour occurs. Organising, as an activity, consists of:

- grouping tasks to achieve objectives
- assigning these tasks
- providing authority, delegating and co-ordinating.

Formal organisation refers to the official network of communication in an organisation, i.e. what the chart shows.

Informal organisation refers to the social hierarchy within working groups and the network of communications between staff in different sections.

The number of levels in an organisation is dependent on size. Smaller organisations tend to have a wider range of duties assigned to individuals, often overlapping. As it grows, so does the need for functional specialisation and a clearer definition of duties and responsibilities. The type of organisation also has an influence – production organisations tend to be flat, and public service organisations tend to be many layered. A clearly structured organisation leads to a clear chain of command within it, which is essential for orderly management.

It is interesting to consider some of the consequences of bad structure. First of all, acquaint yourself with what is considered to be the structure in your workplace.

Draw a picture showing your organisational structure. The ideal may look something like this:

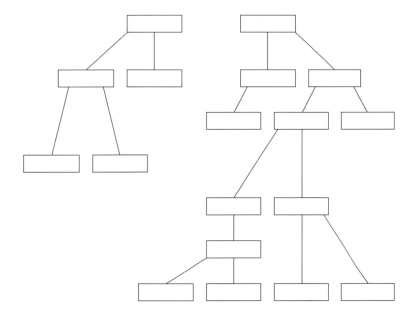

Write in where each staff member belongs. Then draw the reality. What are the consequences of badly designed structure?

Researchers[3] point out there are a number of problems that mark the struggling organisation, all of which can result in rising costs as well as an unhappy workforce. Here are some of the communication failures and their impact on the organisation.

- Inconsistent and arbitrary decisions.
- Poor delegation.

- No job descriptions.
- No appraisal system or formal assessment of performance.
- Poor support systems for managers and supervisors.
- Management not visible and accessible.
- Management information, especially financial, poorly communicated.
- People do not feel free to talk.

Low morale

- Poor communication.
- Lack of relevant, timely information to the right people.
- Failure to re-evaluate past decisions.
- Poor delegation.

Poor decision making

- Conflicting goals.
- Cross purposes.
- Lack of clarity on objectives and priorities.
- Lack of liaison.
- No team working.
- Breakdown between planning and the actual work.

Conflict and lack of co-ordination

Some other symptoms of poor communication are:

- failure to achieve objectives
- low or declining productivity
- high cost of operations and production
- low or declining sales
- high labour turnover
- complaints
- delays in implementing agreed changes
- failure to match competitors
- lack of awareness by managers.

More obvious symptoms of organisational problems are:

- over-manning
- under-manning (mistakes; sickness; high stress)
- delays in making decisions

- managerial disputes
- poor communications.

> **Note which ones feature in your organisation and act quickly to redeem the problem.**

References

1 Welford R and Prescott K (1994) *European Business: an issue-based approach* (2e). Pitman Publishing, London.

2 Mullins LJ (1999) *Management and Organisational Behaviour* (5e). Pitman Publishing, London.

3 Child J (1988) *Organisation: a guide to problems and practice* (2e). Paul Chapman, London.

Further reading

- Handy C (1985) *Understanding Organisations* (2e). Penguin, Harmondsworth.
- Weber M (1964) *The Theory of Social and Economic Organisation*. Collier Macmillan, London.

Part two
The manager's job

CHAPTER 6

The functions of a manager

What is a manager?

Many definitions and views exist but, primarily, managers achieve results through the use of various resources, including people. Management also requires competence in the technical aspects of management, e.g. employment legislation, organisational policy and procedures, quality control, etc.

Management functions are:

- strategic
- tactical
- operational.

The manager's job can be broken down into four main functions:

- planning
- organising
- motivating
- controlling.

Communication and creativity underpin all four functions.

Planning

All levels of management are involved in planning and, to work, these plans must be:

- developed
- long-term
- flexible.

Top management concentrates on overall strategies and long-term plans; what the organisation's goals should be two to ten years ahead.

Middle management concentrates on tactics, i.e. how the overall strategies are to be achieved. This often entails devising and operating short-term plans (from six months to two years ahead).

Supervisors plan work activities, e.g. meeting the month's production quotas. Planning time here varies from a few minutes ahead to a year or even longer.

Planning needs managers who:

- see situations as a whole
- can then break down problems into elements
- are innovative and creative, yet impersonal and analytical when evaluating their ideas
- are quick to spot variances
- have made time for planning.

In planning the managers should aim to make the best use of:

- machinery
- manpower
- materials
- money.

Organising

Organising can mean either:

- working out the actual jobs that need to be done
- giving certain people in the organisation specific jobs to achieve the objectives.

Organising checklist.

- Do you always order material so that the items you need arrive at the most appropriate time?
- Do you communicate your requirements clearly, so that people know exactly what is wanted?
- Do you allocate jobs fairly, balancing skills required against the labour available?
- Do you ensure that every employee is doing their fair share?
- Do you know the capabilities of all employees?

Controlling

Some of the most common misuses of resources in healthcare are:

- overtime

- excessive use of consumables, stationery, cleaning materials etc.
- over or under maintenance
- duplication of effort.

Common failures to reduce costs in general practice are:

- not using all the talents of your workers
- not minimising waiting time
- not using the correct labour – having highly skilled people on routine work
- not having maintenance rotas for equipment, saving expensive repairs or replacements
- not giving staff precise and clear instructions (which help to minimise unnecessary work or mistakes)
- sacrificing quality for quantity
- using the cheapest, but not necessarily the best, material for the job.

These mistakes can be avoided by:

- ordering materials in economic order quantities, well in advance of need
- encouraging staff to be quality minded
- recycling and re-using
- keeping a watch on 'foreigners' – work carried out for the benefit of the worker or one of his friends.

Managers must check frequently to see if they are 'on track' or, if they have fallen short, by how much.

The manager's control function includes controlling costs and waste. The basis for any control system is to keep systematic and specific records, i.e. 'the waste last month was 10.56%' not 'bigger than usual'.

Records should be:

- easy to keep and maintain
- clear and simple to read
- available quickly for inspection
- always up to date.

Functions of a primary care manager

Which level of work do you see yourself doing in your organisation? Senior – strategic, or operational – supervisory. Is this appropriate for you, your skills and your pay? How do your employers see your role?

In early 1993, a group of practice and GP business managers in East Sussex met to discuss their development and training needs. One of the items under discussion was how their employers saw them – their wonder was if GPs saw them as the managers they felt they were, or whether they were viewed as administrators only. This prompted a survey of GPs in East Sussex.

The responses received were varied and interesting and, in part, confirmed the managers' hypothesis that doctors in general practice wanted their managers to be administrators, not managers. However, some wanted these administrators to be very highly trained, up to at least 'A' level, with some requesting a post-graduate qualification.

Eighty-seven percent of the respondents identified their manager as a practice manager, 25% as an administrator, 18% as senior receptionists and 14% as a business/fund manager. These figures did, in part, reflect list size, with smaller, single-handed practices, naming senior administrators, fund holding practices naming business/fund managers. However, when taken in conjunction with the qualifications question, the doctors were expecting quite a lot in terms of qualifications from their senior receptionists.

The majority expected their manager to have taken GCSEs (39%), 30% expected 'A' level standard, 7% degree standard and, surprisingly, 19% wanted a post-graduate qualification. Within this, 10% did not expect a GCSE as a minimum qualification and 19% felt 'A' levels were too high, with a further 33% saying no to a degree level manager.

The conclusion drawn by this group of managers was that, in general, they were managers in name only; the GPs still made all the major decisions, and still refused to hand over total responsibility for management to their managers. The majority of doctor employers interfered in a very disruptive and unconstructive way, and very many confused the decision-making process by being indecisive and not allowing their managers the final say.

It is now 2001. How have things changed? In a recent survey (*Practice Manager*, May 2000) the managers were predominantly white, female (87%), with a mean age of 46.5 years. More than half were educated to 'A' level standard and above and 53% held further management qualifications.

The current role of a practice manager

The practice manager's role has changed considerably over the years and now the NHS is demanding very highly developed management skills. Not all practices have these skills in-house, and some are appointing from outside. The most frequently occurring problem in general practice is that doctors often underestimate the level of management skill required. It is not unusual to find managers appointed from within who have very good organisational and administrative skills but no management experience. Ideally, practice managers need to have this in addition to excellent interpersonal skills, a good level of self-awareness and an ability to research and analyse. Practice managers need to be much more actively involved in strategic and clinical management. For the profession to develop managers need to deliver strategically and to manage, not administrate.

Whoever manages in general practice will have an uneasy task. However well they manage, and however good communications and staff relationships appear, there will always be chaotic pockets.

The manager of the future will need to be able to:[1]

- develop leadership
- drive radical change
- re-shape culture
- exploit the organisation
- keep a competitive edge
- achieve constant renewal
- manage the motivators
- make teamwork work
- achieve total management quality.

Other researchers discuss the keys to management success.

Six keys to success:[2]

Clarity
- Provides clarity in all communications.
- Shows consistency.
- Maintains effective systems for information sharing.

Customers
- Provides a quality service to both staff and customers.

Confidence
- Increases confidence in staff through delegation and continual constructive feedback.
- Acknowledges difficulties and solves problems confidently.
- Seeks new ways of doing things, takes risks.

Co-operation
- Agrees to work in shared ways with staff.
- Team builds.
- Develops and sustains customer relationships.
- Creativity.
- Uses mistakes as learning opportunities.
- Encourages innovation in the team.

Commitment
- Values staff and recognises different talents.
- Ensures staff act responsibly and with accountability.
- Shows commitment to organisational goals.

Choices
- Recognises that s/he can influence outcomes.
- Regards issues not as puzzles with one outcome but examines a range of possible outcomes.
- Transforms problems into opportunities.

Good managers:

- expect results
- develop an atmosphere of encouragement
- give praise, guidance, instructions, constructive criticism
- teach, challenge, stretch their employees
- give more time, are accessible
- encourage questioning and discussion.

Outstanding managers:

- believe in themselves
- have self-confidence
- believe in their own abilities to select, train and teach
- communicate expectations
- believe that employees can learn to make decisions and take initiative.

What is the role of a manager?

The manager has a variety of roles within an organisation. The ones we will concentrate on here are those requiring communicative ability.

- Planning.
- Problem solving.
- Decision-making.
- Networking.
- Co-ordinating.
- Organising.
- Supervising.
- Commanding.
- Controlling.
- Motivating.
- Measuring.
- Communicating.
- Managing conflict.
- Developing staff.
- Disciplining.

For all this they need to have:

- technical competence
- social and human skills
- conceptual ability.

Here are some of the **recommended communication skills** required of today's manager.

- Assertiveness, confidence.
- Excellent verbal and non-verbal communication skills.
- Good interpersonal skills.
- Leadership skills, able to motivate staff.
- Ability to team manage and understand team management.
- Able to act responsibly, working within the limits of his/her own qualification.
- Within known legal and professional boundaries, being accountable for his/her own actions.
- Able to act with integrity, work honestly and conscientiously, respecting the boundaries of confidentiality.
- Able to act in a caring and efficient way, respecting other's needs and individuality, able to listen well.
- Able to retain his/her own professional and personal boundaries, treating colleagues and fellow professionals respectfully and with awareness and integrity.
- Be aware of his/her own ongoing need for professional and personal development.
- Use own initiative.
- Able to discipline and control.

Some of the **key tasks** s/he will be required to do.

- To understand, support and maintain the practice ethos.
- To represent the practice to all professional and public bodies.
- To facilitate consensus between partners, enabling decisions and ensuring they are acted on.
- To support the interests of all groups within the practice.
- To communicate effectively through writing, reading and presentation.
- To be responsible for day-to-day decisions.
- Meetings: preparing, chairing and achieving results.
- Consultation: using internal and external resources.
- Negotiation: formal and internal bargaining.
- Developing people: selection, planning succession, training and developing staff, appraisal, counselling, promotion, managing conflict.
- Managing teams: understanding psychology, motivation and organisational culture.
- Managing change.

- People management: dealing with stress, planning and using time, investing in and supporting staff.
- Taking control: managing the bosses, managing problems, decision-making.
- To co-ordinate, implement and monitor within the practice.
- Strategic management: planning and analysing all aspects of the business and recommending options.
- Selling and marketing: customer relations, prospecting, promoting the business.

Mark off where you, or your manager, meet the above criteria. Look honestly at the gaps and use this to point you in the right direction for training and development. Have you got the skills needed to develop? Do you want to?

Organisational fit

Self-knowledge is invaluable if you are serious about your career development. Using what you have learned so far, ask yourself:

- Is the job right for me?
- What am I good at?
- What type of person am I (a thinker, intuitive, person-centred)?
- What do you value in your job? Power? Achievement? The people?
- Do you plan for the future?
- Does the size and shape of your organisation suit you? What is the corporate image of your organisation? The NHS locally? Globally?
- What are the rules within your organisation – will breaking them be viewed as innovative or non-conformist?
- Are you achieving the right balance between:
    - managing v administrating
    - effectiveness v efficiency
    - overseeing v doing
    - innovating v preserving the status quo?

Effective managers:

- do not just take orders without discussion or challenge
- in discussion with their boss, present their own ideas
- are honest with both the good and bad news
- accept responsibility for their own mistakes or errors of judgement
- praise subordinates when they do well
- take corrective action if required
- ask for advice and help if confused
- delegate
- develop staff.

Effective managers communicate effectively and assertively, in ways that reinforce the self-respect of both parties. See Phillips A (2002) *Assertiveness and the Manager's Job* (Radcliffe Medical Press, Oxford) for ideas on developing these advanced interpersonal and communication skills. The following chapters look in more detail at ways in which managers and others in the practice can improve their communication and interpersonal skills.

References

1   Heller R (1997) *In Search of European Excellence*, Harper Collins Business, London.

2   Sourced from Whitaker V (1994) *Managing People*.

Further reading

- Hunningher E (ed) (1986) *The Manager's Handbook*. Guild Publishing, London.

CHAPTER 7

Problem solving

There is a logical approach to problem solving that most of us, due to pressures of time, do not follow. Every manager needs to set aside time for thinking, planning, and generating solutions to the problems facing them. In this chapter we look at some of the approaches used to assist in solving problems.

Problem solving and decision-making are so inter-related that they are really part of the same process; most problems have a host of possible solutions for which a decision has to be made.

Consider examples of routine decisions that you make every day in your job.

Routine decisions are easy – a definite procedure has been worked out for everyone to follow. They are set by Government legislation, organisational rules or protocols. The most challenging problems are those which are not covered adequately by existing practice or specific rules. Decision-making is one of the cornerstone processes in organisational life – organisational activity consists of a series of decisions. One of the important tasks of a manager is to design appropriate decision-making processes, which is a process made up of several events. What communication and problem solving skills are needed in making decisions?

The **quality** of the decision itself.

- Are appropriate skills and information available?
- Does the organisation have the ability to implement the decision?

The **acceptance** of the decision by the relevant parties involved.

* Everyone in the organisation, especially those in key power positions.
* The people needed to implement it.
* Groups that are important to the organisation – consumers, PCT, professional bodies, etc.

Speed.

* How much time will it take to involve everyone in the decision process?
* If you alter the speed of the process, what might be the cost or benefits in the quality or acceptance of the decision?

Values used in the decision process.

* Define what is good/bad/important/unimportant, in the probable outcome of the decision.
* Decide whose values should be brought to bear on the problems – the manager's?

For example, in locating a new surgery, what weight should be given to employees' desires to live near the surgery? What weight should be given to the community's desire to have car parking versus the local Government public transport policies?

* Who should be involved? At what stage ?
* What importance or weight should be given to their values?

Cost of the decision process.

* What are the monetary and non-monetary costs involved?
* How can the manager identify and evaluate these?

The **flow of events** in the decision process is shown in Figure 7.1.

It is a manager's task to encourage people within the organisation to develop good, creative problem solving skills, and help them in the decision-making process. Encourage them to see around each problem, and generate a host of solutions.

Define the problem. Look through or beyond the problem for the solution. Consider the problem which often occurs at exhibitions, zoos and fairs – children get lost or separated from their parents. If asked to define what the problem is in this type of situation, many respond by saying:

* the problem lies in children getting lost
* the solution lies in reuniting those separated as quickly as possible.

Take a different view; see the problem as one of prevention. The solution then lies in the area of preventing parents and children from being separated in the first place. Or, if a worker suddenly changes his or her behaviour or works badly, consider the situation as more complex than your having a problem with an employee. The problem could be in his/her personal life, relationship with co-workers, or even something you have done.

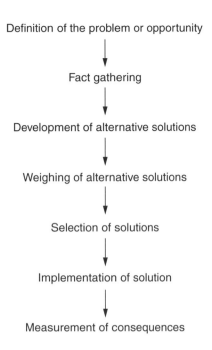

Definition of the problem or opportunity

Fact gathering

Development of alternative solutions

Weighing of alternative solutions

Selection of solutions

Implementation of solution

Measurement of consequences

Figure 7.1   Flow of events

Fact gathering.

- Obtain information.
- Hear all sides of an argument.

Develop **alternative solutions**. There are never any 'right answers' or correct solutions, just a range of alternative courses of action of which one or two are better or more acceptable than the others. To cope with more complex problems we need to be creative as well as logical.

A secretary has tried to free a paper jam in the photocopier, and in the process she has hurt her hand. What courses of action are open?

- Health and safety considerations.
- Established rules and practices.
- Urgency required.
- Cost of implementation.

Select and implement the solution then **measure the consequences**. If the decision is to buy a new piece of machinery, implemention may involve many other aspects, e.g. training, maintenance, cost.

Where a behavioural change is sought, it is important to follow up results.

Solving people problems

People problems are basically concerned with performance. Before these problems can be solved, you need to establish the true nature of the problem by looking at a number of key issues. These will not solve your problems for you, but should tell you what sort of solution you should be looking for. What questions should you ask yourself?

X isn't doing what she should be doing.

- What is the difference in what is being done and what should be done?
- What is it that causes me to say that things are not right?
- Why is this problem important?
- What would happen if I did nothing?
- Is the benefit worth the trouble?
- Is the problem due to a lack of skill or knowledge, or is it something else?
- Could she do it properly if her life depended on it?

If the problem is due to a lack of skill or knowledge then she couldn't do it if her life depended on it.

- Has she ever done the job adequately in the past?
- Has she forgotten through lack of practice?
- Does she have to do this particular task often?
- Does she get regular feedback about how well she does it?
- How does she find out how she is doing?
- Can we change or simplify the job?
- What are the physical and mental qualities needed?
- Could she learn it?

If the problem is not due to a lack of skill or knowledge then it is due to environmental factors.

- Is the required performance punishing?
- What are the consequences to her of doing the job properly?
- Is non-performance self-rewarding?
- What are the consequences for her of doing it her way rather than mine?
- What does she get out of her performance in terms of rewards, status, prestige?
- Does she get more attention by doing it wrong than doing it right?
- Does performance matter to her?
- Can she expect a favourable outcome for doing it right, or an unfavourable one for doing it wrong?
- What are the obstacles to her performance?
- Does she know what is expected of her?

- Has she got the authority, the time, the tools and the information needed to do the job properly?
- Is it an impossible job anyway?

Making decisions

- *State aims*: identify the essential and desirable aims of the decision.
- *Search for alternatives*: using brainstorming.
- *Evaluate the alternatives*: by using a risk analysis, financial or time evaluation, or feasibility study.
- *Assess the consequences*: to employees and partners, the environment and other people.

Only then do you take a personal decision on the best course of action. At this point you implement the decision by planning the change, and involving people.

- Schedule what has to be done, by whom and when. Use memos, discussions, charts, meetings, training sessions.
- Recognise what is going on during your interactions with people singly or in a group, and how this affects your decision-making. Is your leadership effective? Was conflict handled well? How can individuals be helped to participate?

Another way to help you make a decision is to weigh up the pros and cons of a prospective change. Use a chart to measure and thus clarify your thoughts.

This chart looks at a decision-making process for moving to the country. Weight your answers, with a score of ten as positive and zero as negative.

	Village	*Market town*	*Isolated cottage*
Isolation	5	10	0
Dependence on car	5	10	0
Good amenities	3	8	0
Anonymity	1	10	7
Peace and quiet	8	5	10
TOTALS	22 = 2nd	**43 = 1st**	17 = 3rd

The logical approach

Other problem solving techniques

Although most of us, in the course of living, develop a characteristic way of coping with difficulties – trial and error, careful analysis, intuition – few of us possess a repertoire of problem solving techniques. The following sets out examples of fairly simple but widely used techniques which can be utilised either collectively or individually in the workplace. Managers will play a key role in initiating or co-ordinating the thought process.

SWOT analysis

Consider the strengths and weaknesses, and opportunities and threats within the problem. The following brief example demonstrates the analysis with a practice considering an individual PMS contract.

- Strengths:
  - Committed partnerships.
  - Good financial management.
  - Computerised for four years.
  - High quality practice manager.
- Weaknesses:
  - Insufficient room in premises.
  - Lack of consistency in approach between partners in referrals and prescribing.
  - Time management.
- Opportunities:
  - Reduce waiting lists.
  - Improve quality of care offered.
  - Improve quality of local services.
- Threats:
  - Practice manager leaves.
  - To income.
  - To pensions.

The six step approach

Analyse the problem.

- Does the problem exist?
- Define it – set out what needs to be understood.
- What is the cause?

Decide on a solution.

- Generate alternatives, link ideas.
- Evaluate, test, and select one.
- Implement the change and follow up.

Use a chart

The problem is	The problem is not	Distinctive features	Who or what is involved
What Automatic sensor – doors open/close by themselves	Any other type of malfunction		Patients confused!
Where Only downstairs			
When Late afternoon/ early evening		Seems to be connected to putting telephone over to deputising service	
Who to contact	Company BT Insurers Put a note up for patients		

Analysing

There is a need for careful analysis before embarking on the decision-making process. You need to:

- *Recognise the problem*: you know there is a problem when the standard you have fixed is not being attained. However, standards are assumed, they may be historic and inherited, or made by your own judgement. Is there a problem?
- *Specify it*: record what/when/where it is and what it isn't, how big is it and does it change with time?
- *Collect information*: again – who, why, what and where from? Is the information you have been given accurate? What are the interests and biases of your informants?
- *Identify the causes*: decide what problems could have caused this one – brainstorm or create a problem tree, use your own ideas and others' experiences.
- *Test the causes*: ascertain whether the cause identified could have accounted for the whole problem.

To simplify:

Problem	Solution	Positives (+)	Negatives (−)	Action

Problem solving checklist

Review the current process for getting blood samples analysed at your practice, for example:

- Highlight the **benefits** which could accrue from analysing tests in the surgery.
- Identify areas of **additional costs**.
- Assuming the benefits make the machine a viable development, list the **changes** to the surgery you would expect and a **timetable** for implementation.
- Consider the pros and cons of a **trial period** and patient satisfaction.
- **Implement** and **review**.

Every service uses resources (staff time, equipment, etc) and these resources have to be used effectively. A timetable for implementation will ensure that a proposed development occurs in a logical and systematic way. A review mechanism allows the practice to assess the effectiveness of change and fine tune service provisions.

Detail an **action plan** with **timetable**. **Allocate action** to different members of the team. **Review.**

The creative approach

Find out:

- how, where, what, and/or how specifically does this problem occur?
- when it became a problem?
- why it is important
- if there was a time when it wasn't a problem and, if so, what is different now?
- what solutions you have already applied.

Explore the solution space.

- Give at least three possible solutions to the problem.
- Which one jumps out at you as being the most feasible?
- How will you know when the problem is solved?
- What would be the first step to making that a reality?
- When and where are you going to take that step?

Use a soft systems approach[1] and draw a picture (called a Rich picture), which shows how you see the problem. This helps both to identify and analyse problems in complex, and confusing, settings – like general practice.

- Write down any solutions that, in retrospect, you feel would work.
- Write down those that you would not consider.
- Are there any left over that you are not sure about? Do not dismiss them. Make a note of them and come back to them at a later date.
- Write or draw the consequences of some of the solutions you are considering.

Identify the problems as 'messes' (unmanageable, impossible to untangle, unsolvable, and tend not to have clear boundaries) or 'difficulties' (smaller, with less people involved, with limited implications and likely solutions known). These may be treated separately, with clearer priority.

Reversal

Dr Edward de Bono, director of the Cognitive Research Trust at Cambridge, illustrates this technique with the problem of an ambulance which, rushing along a narrow voluntary road, comes up behind a flock of sheep. To try to get the ambulance past the sheep would be slow, and might harm the sheep. So, get the sheep past the ambulance – stop the vehicle, turn the flock round and lead it back past the stationary ambulance.

Redefinition

The solution to a problem often depends on the way it is stated. If you define it narrowly you open up a range of possibilities. You have one car and four drivers – don't ask 'How can we make the car available to whoever needs it?' Instead, try – 'How can we meet our needs without using the car?' Join a car pool. Use bicycles. Time and stagger the car use.

Planning for results

This technique is based on the conviction that what looks like a problem will solve itself. Outline expected results and work backwards. An answer to 'How can the practice agree on what to do with a financial windfall?' would not begin with Dr A's longing for a new autoclave, or the reception's campaign for a new telephone system. Instead, the question would be: 'What does this practice want for itself five or ten years from now? What action should be taken now, or later, to promote this outcome?' Once the goal has been defined, the problem is half solved.

Breaking routines

For example, if you work nights and rarely get to eat a main meal with your family, rearrange your schedule so that the whole family share a substantial meal at breakfast time, and have sandwiches for supper. The new routine will cut down your cooking time and give your children a chance to be with you.

Brainstorming

This popular technique:

- involves everyone
- is non-threatening
- encourages communication and creativity
- maximises solutions to problems
- minimises the risk of overlooking elements of the problem.

If some of the questions or answers provoke strong feelings, give space for these to be aired. Don't bury them! If you are working this through in a team, expect tensions, arguments and difficulties. Everyone will have a different agenda.

- Feelings often produce more creative solutions to problems.
- Being there can be enough, you do not have to solve the problem.
- Empathise so the problem is shared.
- Create a safe, confidential space to air any conflicts.
- Prioritise doubts and uncertainties.
- Allow and encourage conflict.
- Tolerate criticism directed at you.
- Support those less socially skilled.
- Learning is best achieved by honest sharing.
- Be prepared to take risks.

When you want to generate a lot of ideas quickly to solve problems, use the following brainstorming techniques.

- Work in a small group of six to ten people.
- Sit in a semi-circle or a U-shape.
- Appoint someone from the group to record the ideas on a flip chart.
- As the ideas are recorded and the flip chart sheets are filled, they are then torn off and taped across the front of the room.
- No criticism or evaluation is allowed during a session. Comments like 'that's ridiculous' cool enthusiasm, and lead individuals to defend rather than generate ideas. In a non-judgemental atmosphere, people feel free to contribute whatever comes into their minds in the way of solutions. In turn, these ideas give rise to more ideas.
- Encourage participants to think of the wildest ideas. It's easier to tone down than to think up.

- Emphasis is on quantity, not quality. The more ideas produced, the more good ideas are likely to turn up.
- Participants are urged to build upon or modify each other's ideas.
- When the given time is up, the group discusses the ideas and chooses the top three or four to consider further.
- After the group has had time to think about the ideas, a second meeting is called for more discussion and a vote.

Here is what a family came up with during a ten-minute session on how to cut food costs.

- Give up desserts.
- Experiment with eggs, dried peas or beans as a meat substitute.
- Persuade everyone to diet or fast one day a week.
- Join a bulk-buying group.
- Plant a garden.
- Buy in larger quantities.
- Set a per-serving cost limit and stick to it.
- Offer smaller helpings.

You can brainstorm by yourself. Write down everything that occurs to you, then put the list aside. When you pick it up again, you may find the solution to your problem.

Making a minus a plus

The heart of many problems lies in what seems to be a single, intractable element. When that's the case, don't ask, 'How can I minimise this liability?' but 'How can I make the most of it?'

When you have a good product with an apparent drawback – an effective children's play area, say, that looks old fashioned and unattractive – don't try to conceal the liability. Exaggerate it, present it as something special, paint it bright red and attach silver discs, then the minus becomes a plus.

A young woman, just embarking on a career as a NHS manager, had set her sights on a job with a prestigious local practice, but everyone urged her to get experience at a smaller practice first. No seriously big practice, they insisted, would hire an untried new graduate. Nevertheless, she applied to her chosen practice. Asked about her experience, she said, 'None at all, but I want to learn this business with a top-quality practice. Hire me and you can train me to suit your needs. I won't have to unlearn faulty techniques acquired elsewhere.' She got the job.

Reference

1   Checkland P (1999) *Systems Thinking, Systems Practice*. Wiley, Chichester.

CHAPTER 8

Leadership skills

All managers have their own, individual, way of leading.

Are you a good leader?

Can you see yourself in the following list? Are you someone who:

- solves problems creatively
- communicates and listens well
- hopes to achieve
- has many interests
- respects and believes in their subordinates
- has self-confidence and enthusiasm
- has self-discipline and is emotionally stable.

New and more robust leadership will be expected if primary care is going to lead within the NHS. This chapter addresses the sorts of skills required to enable this.

Some problems with leadership in general practice.

- Poor leadership structures and unclear lines of accountability weaken the structure.
- It is often unclear who the leader is, with the staff **responsible** to the manager, but **accountable** to the partners. Uncertainty and confusion sets in as management is undermined.
- If old fashioned partners head up the practice, it will tend to lead with a predominantly autocratic, task orientated style.
- Managers function to personify the organisation, but too often serve as a scapegoat when things go wrong.
- Managers may have little influence over either activities within the organisation or the outcomes.
- Managers are often appointed to a position of leadership. They accept an **image** of personal control without the authority to control.
- Other people in the organisation often act as (unpaid and unacknowledged) leaders. Once people assume power, they are unconsciously given it.

The leader need not necessarily be the manager – in fact within general practice there is often a need for the partners to lead, and for the manager to **enable** this to happen, by co-ordinating the change required. The leader visions, the manager controls. There is a shift occurring in some practices, with some of the younger partners looking to share the control, moving their organisations toward a more modern, participative and supportive management style; they see the more structured style of management as having too many attendant difficulties.

Office politics and power games are played out in all large and small organisations – people jockey for position, hold grudges, have petty jealousies and rivalries. The most negative of human emotions are displayed because we are human, and we will all, at some time or another, act out our distresses. The practice manager will be expected to 'hold' or contain these tensions, and work with and around them in order to minimise their harmful impact. This is a tough job, and one that needs skill and patience.

There are several ways to manage, but most people adopt a style that they feel comfortable with and which matches the expectations of the people they work for. Most move through a matrix of styles depending on the situation facing them. They move fluidly, unconsciously, sometimes finding themselves behaving autocratically when their style is usually democratic, but more often adopting styles consciously depending on the situation. For example, there is a need to be autocratic at times of rapid and imposed change or crisis – someone has to make decisions fast. A more diplomatic stance can be adopted when there is the time to consult and debate. Each style carries its own strengths and weaknesses and the reader will recognise their own approach. To recap on some of the most common approaches, are you:

- **Autocratic?**
- **Bureaucratic?**
- **Diplomatic?**
- **Free-rein?**
- **Participative?**

Some notes on different leadership styles.

- Supportive leadership is related to lower staff turnover, less grievance rates and better staff satisfaction, and results in less inter-group conflict.
- Directive leadership increases productivity, but only if the task is routine and repetitive. This may work with simple tasks such as database operation, or administrative tasks.
- Structured leadership – where the manager leads – is usually the most productive style when managing a crisis.
- Autocratic leadership leads to an equally powerful force within the practice – resisting management, wanting to be managed, but not knowing by whom or how. In this scenario other people within the practice

make formal or informal bids for leadership at different times, which complicates matters. There are clear implications for action, but action can only succeed personal learning.

One of the ways you can measure the happiness and healthiness of your organisation is to look at some of the key issues to staff satisfaction.

- Good communication.
- Democratic leadership.
- Leaders promote innovation.
- Staff are consulted.
- Training and development needs are met.
- Team or group working occurs.
- Motivational needs are met.
- Culture is understood.

Researchers reporting in the *Health Service Journal*[1] have found that staff want:

- genuine interest in their individuality
- a view through their eyes
- leaders to value their contributions and develop their strengths
- leaders to have positive expectations of staff.

The best leaders, they felt were:

- inspirational communicators, networkers and achievers
- empowering
- transparent
- accessible, approachable and flexible
- decisive, determined, ready to take risks
- able to draw people together with a shared vision
- charismatic
- able to challenge the status quo
- able to analyse and think creatively
- able to manage change sensitively and skilfully.

Practices can only achieve by the co-ordinated efforts of their members, and it is the manager's task to get work done through other people. Thus the manager must understand the nature of leadership.

Here are some thoughts on leadership.

- Leadership skills can be learned and developed.
- Leadership transforms the performance of the organisation.
- Leadership style has an effect on those led.

Where leadership is top driven, command and control are the keywords and the power base is determined by the owner or managers.[2] Now that the primary care brief is widening it is becoming more common to find people working in a situation where the power base is held by expert teams, not individuals – people who work collectively on clearly defined subject areas. This is a more modern and popular way of working.

Of course, working within a clearly defined autocratic, hierarchical and bureaucratic organisation has its benefits. Staff know where they sit, their responsibilities are clearly defined, and change is easy to impose. However, it is not a modern or popular way of working, it rarely uses all the skills within the organisation, and it is not good for staff morale. Younger staff in particular now demand and expect to work more flexibly, and have their ideas, wishes and responses listened to and acted on more tolerably. Hierarchical working also breeds discriminatory practice as it only incorporates a one-sided idea (the bosses') of correctness, standards and principles. In successful organisations devolved responsibilities mean the power base is held by expert teams, not individuals; staff work collectively to problem solve defined subject areas. This way of working should be encouraged as it paves the way for flexible, innovative working.

Look critically at your practice.

- Is your leadership style relaxed and accommodating?
- Are you proactive?
- Is leadership top-driven?
- Is the power base determined by the owner/managers?
- Do people work collectively?
- Do staff understand their responsibilities?
- Is change easy to impose?
- Do staff work flexibly?
- Do people have their ideas, wishes and responses listened to and acted upon?
- Do you promote innovation and creativity?

Team working takes time. People strapped for time make decisions alone. There is no time to consult. This directive and controlling model results in policies being adhered to, but in some areas compliance is not good, and staff are unhappy. The approach clearly determines the way staff may be expected to fit in with the organisational objectives. It is designed to make unilateral management action more palatable. Senior management decide the overall strategy and plan – and nobody else is involved.

Simplistic models of people management seek to direct and control, and see people as dispensable. Best practice shows us organisations where the decision-making is devolved down, and ideas are fed up. The use of 'quality groups' demonstrates good employee involvement (as recommended in the 'excellence' literature).[3] Here a series of workplace groups are set up to initiate and develop workplace initiatives. Responsibility for creativity and ideas is devolved down, so everyone in the organisation has responsibility for being part of the decision-making process. Change, initiative, and learning through trial and error are then not feared but viewed positively. People are encouraged by being involved, and directing the agenda for change.

Practice managers need to lead their organisation towards the leading edge of change, by shifting from a simple, perhaps bureaucratic, structure to a more complex, mature organisational approach to human resource management:

Does your organisation:

- devolve decision-making?
- feed up ideas?
- use 'quality groups'?
- encourage creativity, initiative, learning?
- encourage employee involvement?
- encourage the habits of self-discipline and initiative?

The manager as an enabler

Clearly, it is advantageous for the manager to empower his or her staff to enable them to feel comfortable and confident enough to make crucial and responsible decisions by themselves, without constant recourse to someone more senior.

Changing leadership styles

If practices need to change their present style of leadership, the benefits to the organisation are:

- financial (the practice could grow into the role expected of it)
- organisational (less conflict for those working within the organisation)
- personal (less stress).

However, change is painful and difficult, and needs to be managed well for everyone to be comfortable with the process. Practices need to be especially aware of the 'Change Management Transition Curve', and to offer support through the attendant mourning process. In this process, people go through a period of denial and resistance to change, followed by commitment to the change and a degree of exploration towards the future. Managers need to be aware of the beliefs that inform individual resistance to change, so they can work with, rather than against, the resistance. (For more information on change management, see Phillips A (2002) *Assertiveness and the Manager's Job*. Radcliffe Medical Press, Oxford.)

Some larger organisations are now too big for their managers to manage everything successfully and sensitively – there are too many time pressures that lead to an autocratic style of management, even if the preferred style, at less stressful times, might be more enabling. If this is the case, it may be best for the practice to take time out to review the management role, by involving the whole team, looking at those tasks that can be taken on by other leaders in the organisation. Whatever decisions are made, it is imperative that the whole organisation is involved at whatever level, and for everyone to be clear about those decisions.

Leadership v management

Fundamentally, leadership is about being able to influence the behaviour of others. A leader is someone who achieves results through people. Leaders are not born; we all have the potential to lead but there's no gift of leadership. Every leader has to make their own way. All managers are leaders, but paradoxically, not all leaders are managers.

Leader behaviour is influenced by:

- personality
- the task in hand (is it structured or unstructured?)
- the organisational culture
- the team being handled.

Some points about leadership.

- A good leader understands his/her own style.
- S/he can diagnose the degree of control needed in each situation.
- S/he can change to suit.
- Leadership is easier if the team has similar personality attributes in training, experience, age, sex or other personal characteristics – this is less threatening to the leader.
- It is easier if you like your team!

What kind of leadership behaviour do you see in yourself?

Are you:

- task orientated: directive, concerned with guiding, directing, standards and performance?
- achievement and goal orientated: wanting people to strive to perform?
- person orientated: participative, wanting to empower your team?
- supportive: wanting to compensate for what you see as difficult conditions?

Many years of solid research in health, education and industry have demonstrated clearly that the choice of leadership style should depend on the situation.

- The job to be done.
- How important it is to attend to the people doing the job (by maintaining morale, for example).
- The motivation of your employees – their education, experience and willingness to work alone.

Different styles of leadership are appropriate for different stages of a business[4]:

Where is your business?	Skills needed
A new venture	Team driving
	To provide wide range of management skill
	To have innovation and energy
Entering growth stage	Manager to develop strong, supportive team
	Driving leadership qualities
Mature. Meeting boundaries erected by competitors	To ensure efficiency and economy
	Planning skills
	Cost control
	Sound personnel policies
Premature decline	Tough and innovative
	Cut costs
	Improve productivity
	Reduce staffing levels

The realities that shape our choice of role are:

- what the organisation expects of us
- what is defined as a suitable style.

In general practice a laid back, democratic leadership style is often less threatening to the doctors; in larger health organisations a sharper approach is preferred.

Look at the advantages and disadvantages of the following leadership styles:

The prescriber
- Plans, informs, tells, rules.
- Prescribes and directs.
- Makes decisions alone.
- Uses one-way communication.
- Frequently checks on the progress.
- Minimises personal interactions.
- Expects compliance.

In times of crisis the talented solo leader is effective in overcoming barriers and implementing decisions. However, when these leaders fail, they are discarded. The style encourages staff not to take responsibility for their actions – the problems are passed up to someone more senior to solve. It is not an empowering leadership style.

Questions to ask yourself if you are a prescriber.

- Do I have enough information to make a good decision?
- If I were to make the decision by myself, would it be accepted?
- Is acceptance by staff critical to effective implementation?

The persuader
- Persuades people to do the job.
- Sets standards, provides support and encouragement.
- Treats people as equals.
- Invites two-way communication.
- Interacts socially.

Questions to ask yourself if you are a persuader.

- Have you obtained agreement to do the job?
- Have you spent time getting to understand your team's problem?
- Have you tried to help solve them?

The participator
- Is a coach to a group of professionals.
- Encourages people to solve the problems themselves, assisting only when they ask for help.
- Acts as a consultant.
- Shares the problem, but ultimately makes the decision.

Questions to ask yourself if you are a participator.

- Who would you use this style with?
- Have you communicated general expectations about methods and results?

The permitter
- Gives very little direction.
- Provides a general definition of the job.

- Allows people to provide their own structure.
- Deliberately restricts their role, provides limited help and support.
- Creates a sense of mission.
- Acts as a chair, for the group to reach consensus.
- Accepts and implements the solution, which the group supports.

Managers acting to support a group of clinicians in their clinical decision would use this style. When used with subordinates, it is very empowering, respectful, and trusting.

Questions to ask yourself if you are a permitter.

- Can staff be trusted to base solutions on organisational considerations?
- Do they have sufficient additional information to result in a high quality decision?

Do you tell or sell? Participate or delegate?

Leadership and control

Research suggests[5] that the manner and amount of **control** that is exercised in an organisation has an effect on employee performance (*see* Figure 8.1). Any management system that controls must take into account:

- the individuals concerned
- social factors
- organisational factors.

These determine people's psychology. Leaders need to be aware of the forces in the manager, in the people they manage, the situation being managed, and the pressures of time.

- Control provides either a safe or constraining boundary.
- Control either restricts or gives freedom of choice.
- Control implies something about the individual's standing within the organisation.
- People feel good and powerful when they exercise control.
- The exercise of control helps individuals identify with their workplace.
- People who exercise control may be more willing to conform.

However:

- there will always be resistance to control from those people with low self-esteem and less belief in authority.

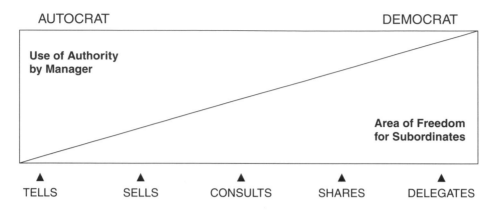

Figure 8.1   Continuum of leadership behaviour [5]

Some important principles

Leadership is about sharp interpersonal communication skills. It is about achieving results through people, by being:

* sensitive to their wants
* recognising of their needs
* inspiring in your ideas
* authentic in your actions.

Good leaders recognise the needs of those they lead. People need:

* to be heard
* to be understood
* to be recognised
* to be respected
* to be rewarded
* to be motivated
* to achieve.

You can be a more effective leader by developing yourself.

* Develop your sensitivity.
* Develop your awareness.
* Develop your creativity.
* Organise your time better.
* Improve your communication skills.

Develop your team – the more effective the people you manage are, the better your management skills will be perceived.

* Delegate.
* Coach.

- Mentor.
- Counsel.
- Train.

References

1 Alimo-Metcalfe B and Alban-Metcalfe R (2000) Leadership. *HSJ*. **October 12**: 26–8.

2 Mintzberg H (1973) *The Nature of Managerial Work*. Harper and Row, New York.

3 Peters TJ and Waterman RH (1982) *In Search of Excellence*. Harper and Row, London.

4 Clark C and Pratt S (1985) Leadership's four-part progress. *Management Today*.

5 Adapted from Tannenbaum R and Schmidt WH (1973) How to choose a leadership pattern. *Harvard Business Review*. **May/June**: 162–75, 178–80.

Further reading

- Belbin RM (1993) *Team Roles at Work*. Butterworth-Heinemann, Oxford.
- Handy C (1993) *Understanding Organisations* (4e). Penguin Books, Harmondsworth.
- McGregor D (1987) *The Human Side of Enterprise*. Penguin, Harmondsworth.
- Mullins LJ (1999) *Management and Organisational Behaviour* (5e). Pitman, London.
- Vroom V and Yetton P (1973) *Leadership and Decision-Making*. University of Pittsburgh Press.

CHAPTER 9

Delegation

Delegation is crucial in any place of work. Doctors, chief executives, directors, managers, supervisors, all have a responsibility to delegate some of their work so that they can concentrate on those tasks that only they are best able to, and paid to, do. It is very common in general practice to find poor patterns of delegation – it is an underused art.

Why is it so hard to delegate?

Although it is relatively easy to get people to agree that delegation is worthwhile, many do not delegate as effectively as they could. There are reasons for this, find which one speaks for you:

- *You manage your own time badly, you are overstretched and spend time doing instead of planning.* Busy practices are working to capacity. Distinguish between the urgent things and the important things. Delegation leaves you free to give attention to more important matters.
- *Your responsibilities and limit of authority are not clear to you, or anyone else in the practice.* If you are uncertain about this you simply cannot delegate effectively. Become certain. Find out.
- *You underestimate the competence of your subordinates and genuinely believe that you can do the work better than anyone else.* This may be true but it does not follow that you will get as much done as a properly co-ordinated work team. As we climb within our own hierarchy, the strategic content of the job increases as the operational, 'doing' content declines. We cannot hope to remain specialists with superior technical skills after moving into a job which has quite different requirements. Inadequate subordinates will never improve if you do their work for them. They must either be moved or developed (by delegation).
- *You feel threatened by the competence of your subordinates.* Do some more work to raise your self-esteem, and develop a more secure sense of self.
- *You feel insecure in your job and in your work relationships.* If delegation is the right to make decisions, then it must include the right to make

mistakes too, for anyone who makes decisions will inevitably make a mistake at some time. How big a mistake are you willing to let someone else make? Many managers fail to delegate because they fear the criticism if a mistake is made. To delegate properly, you must be confident that you can solve any problem which your subordinates may create. Delegation is not abdication.

People who feel insecure in their positions make poor delegators for a variety of reasons.

* They may be afraid of not being essential.
* They may feel more competent and comfortable performing routine duties instead of the work of a manager – planning, organising, controlling, and leading.
* They do not want to appear lazy to their seniors, colleagues and subordinates, or even to themselves.

Having identified the reasons why you do not delegate, let us examine some of the principles of delegation.

The principles of delegation

There is no absolute rule as to the number that one person can effectively manage. This depends on:

* the nature of work
* ability/training of subordinates
* the degree of delegation
* the degree of communication distance.

It also depends on who carries the following responsibilities:

* **Authority**: who has the right and legitimate power to delegate responsibility?
* **Responsibility**: involves an obligation by the subordinate to perform certain duties.
* **Accountability**: who carries ultimate responsibility?

Delegating is entrusting responsibility and authority to others (not necessarily just subordinates) who then become **responsible** to you for results. The delegator remains **accountable** for the performance of their subordinates. What you delegate essentially is the right to make decisions. Authority and responsibility go hand in hand. A person cannot be responsible for a task if authority to act is not given. One can never avoid responsibility by delegation – 'passing the buck'.

Delegation is the process by which a manager grants or permits the transfer of authority to someone to operate within prescribed limits. Whoever delegates has to have the permission within the organisation to do so.

The main stages in the process of delegation are:

- clarifying objectives
- agreeing the terms of reference, authority and responsibility
- guidance, support and training
- agreement on monitoring and review periods
- allowing freedom of action with agreed terms of reference
- rewarding.

The principles of delegation are to:

- establish reasonable objectives
- offer definite training and instructions
- be accessible
- monitor
- share thinking and objectives to provide a background for subordinates' decisions
- let them know what is expected of them and how results will be evaluated.

Why delegate?

- Good delegation gives you more time for thinking and planning – and taking the big decisions that cannot be delegated.
- The person closest to the activity should be better able to make decisions.
- Delegation tends to encourage initiative, which, in turn, improves morale.
- Delegation equips people to solve their own problems.
- Delegation reduces decision time.
- People enhance their contribution to the organisation by concentrating on tasks to which they are best suited.
- Good delegation makes you dispensable – and that should help your promotion chances.

Prerequisites for delegation.

- The development of organisation objectives, policies and guidelines.
- Clear definitions of the responsibilities and authority of each job, in writing. This provides greater freedom than ambiguous or inconsistent boundaries.
- Time schedule, identification of specific results and means of measurement.
- The specific roles of both the delegator and those delegated to.
- Provision for control and minimum time between feedback and correction of deviations.

Five levels of delegation. The 'delegatee':

- investigates and reports back
- investigates and recommends action
- investigates and advises of intended action
- investigates and takes action; advises of action taken
- investigates and takes action.

Which bird of delegation are you?[1]

- **The White-Shirted Hoverer** – a bird who gives a subordinate a job to do and then perches on their shoulder.
- **The Pin-Striped Whoopster** – a bird who watches closely over their subordinates and becomes very raucous when they deviate from the way they think the job should be done.
- **The Yellow-Bellied Credit Snatcher** – a bird well known and often highly regarded.
- **The Lesser White-Crested Cuckoo** – the bird who, by habit, lays their eggs in the other's nest.
- **The Duck-Billed Double-Talker** – a bird who really never made clear what authority they meant to delegate.
- **The Golden-Crowned Mourning Dope** – a bird who mourns the lack of people they can trust with decisions, yet who won't let anyone else decide anything.
- **The Black and White Organisation Creeper** – the bird who delegates authority and then creeps around the structure to lower level subordinates and thereby nullifies the delegation.
- **The Redheaded Firefighter** – who thinks they are delegating authority when they ask their subordinates to check with them before making even the most minor decisions.
- **The Lion-Kicking Vulture** – sits back and waits for their subordinates to make important mistakes and then kicks these 'dead lions' with gusto and bravado.

When and what to delegate

What to delegate.
In general, the subordinate should tackle predictable tasks, while the more experienced should handle exceptional ones. These types of tasks should be delegated down:

- Matters that keep repeating themselves.
- Minor decisions most frequently made.
- Details that take the biggest chunks of time.
- Parts of the job the superior is least qualified to handle.

- Job details the superior most dislikes.
- Parts of the job that make the superior overspecialised.

What not to delegate – any key management roles.

- Setting objectives: these are the responsibility of management.
- Organising employees into an efficient team.
- Motivation and communication.
- Checking and analysing results: part of the control function.
- Developing subordinate skills in routine decision-making: delegating is a managerial responsibility.
- The things that only you can do:
  - Overall policy for your department.
  - Overall planning.
  - Selection, training and appraisal of your immediate subordinates.
  - Promotion, praise and disciplinary action for your immediate subordinates.
- Final accountability for the work of your department.
- Anything to people not capable of doing the work effectively or to people who do not work for you.

In summary, do delegate:

- anything someone can do **better, quicker, cheaper** than or **instead** of, you.

Do not delegate:

- confidential matters
- legally/contractually restricted jobs
- disciplinary actions
- ultimate accountability.

When to delegate.

- Let your own subordinates control their work, even if, to begin with, they do not handle things quite as well as you do. Remember that each job should be tackled at the lowest possible level.
- Delegate as a contribution to staff training and development. If you feel you cannot trust a subordinate with a job, then train them.
- Delegate to assess suitability for promotion.

See Appendix A for some exercises to see if you delegate fairly and competently, and have planned for your succession.

Making it easier to delegate

1   Be sure you and your boss agree on what your job is.
2   Be sure your subordinates understand what you expect them to do.

* **Agree** the area of his/her responsibility and the required standards of performance.
* **Give them the means** of carrying out their task: authority, knowledge, the materials, people and preferably a budget.
* **Specify objectives** in qualitative terms with a target date for completion – but allow your subordinate to choose their own methods.
* **Let them make their own decisions,** with guidance whenever requested, subject to periodic checks and feedback.
* **Build up confidence** by resisting the desire to over-criticise if a mistake is made.
* **Discourage subordinates from 'half-taking' decisions** and leaving the rest to you – get them to think problems right through and act on their judgement.
* **Set up a control system** so that you can correct deviations from agreed standards.
* **Reward** the people who get things done. People will accept responsibility and actively participate in accomplishing the objectives of the organisation only if they feel that rewards go to the people who get things done. The rewards for being right must always be greater than the penalties for being wrong. These rewards will include knowledge of results, promotion, pay, a friendly chat, respect and so on.

Use delegation as a means of developing subordinates.

* **Review** every six months and discuss overall performance.
* **Say** how well the objectives agreed have been achieved and what could be done to improve. Suggest suitable objectives for the next six months, and ways in which the job might change in the future.
* **Listen to their views** on the problems encountered in working towards their objectives, whether they now think the objectives were unrealistic, ways in which you could have helped more, ways in which they think the job has changed, and where they want to go from here.
* **Agree** on what the job is, and what you are trying to achieve. Agree on what you are each going to do in the next six months.

If you are having problems with delegation, check whether you are taking advantage of key people with more knowledge and experience than you in certain aspects of the work – in terms of time (because they are on the spot) or salary costs (because they are paid less).

The less than ideal solution at the right time may be far better than the otherwise ideal solution at the wrong time.

Setting objectives

Those delegating need to be clear about the aims and objectives of the job they are delegating. Objectives should:

- be brief, yet cover the main features of the job
- be verifiable
- state the time when they are to be achieved
- indicate the quality of objectives and the cost of achieving them
- present a challenge
- indicate priorities.

Criteria for good objectives.

- Do they indicate:
  - quantity (how much)?
  - quality (how well, or specific characteristics)?
  - time (when)?
  - cost (at what cost)?
  - if qualitative in nature, are objectives nonetheless verifiable?
- Are the objectives challenging, yet reasonable?
- Are priorities assigned to the objective (ranking, weighting, etc.)?
- Are the objectives co-ordinated with other departments? Are they consistent with the objectives of the superior, the practice, the NHS as a whole?
- Are they communicated to all who need to be informed?
- Are the assumptions underlying the objectives clearly identified?
- Are the objectives expressed clearly and in writing?
- Do the objectives provide for timely feedback so that any necessary corrective steps can be taken?
- Are the resources and authority sufficient for achieving the objectives?
- Have the individuals who are expected to accomplish objectives been given a chance to suggest their own?
- Does the individual have control over aspects for which he or she is assigned responsibility?

Additional delegation hints.

- Use mistakes for learning.
- Rotate jobs.
- Don't overload high achievers.
- Encourage questions.

See the Appendix for some delegation dilemmas.

References

1 Sourced from Supervisor's Pack (1997) Brighton College of Technology, Brighton.

2 Fred Pryor Seminars (1997) *Delegation Dilemmas*. Pryor Resources Inc., Shawnee Mission Parkway.

Further reading

* Mullins LJ (1999) *Management and Organisational Behaviour* (5e). Pitman Publishing, London.

Appendix

Exercise 1. Can you delegate fairly and competently, and have you planned for your succession?

- Draw up a list of the job responsibilities you would leave behind if you were to suddenly leave your practice.
- List the subordinates qualified to take over each of those responsibilities. If there is no-one available, leave a blank.
- Give each blank one of the following reasons:
  - inadequate subordinate (for whatever reason)
  - poorly defined management structure
  - your choice (for whatever reason).
- Make a list of duties which you could delegate but don't. Work out why you don't.
- If appropriate, make a list of duties that could be delegated to you. Establish why this has not happened.

Exercise 2. How well do you delegate?

- Are decisions in your organisation made at the lowest level at which they can properly be made?
- Do your subordinates know what you expect them to do?
- Do your subordinates have policies to guide them in making decisions?
- Is your department organised in a way that facilitates delegation?
- Do you direct your subordinates to accomplish certain results, or simply to perform certain activities?
- Do you make the fullest possible use of your staff?
- Do you spend enough time on the really important parts of your job?
- Do you spend too much time 'putting out fires' – dealing with constant emergencies demanding your personal attention which keep you from working on the major issues?
- Does your work face constant deadline crises, with some dates missed and others only just 'getting under the wire'?
- Do you regularly take work home or stay late in the office?
- Do you yield to the temptation to take your coat off and do the job yourself?
- Ask yourself what should I be doing and what should I not be doing.
- Ask yourself how can I best equip each of my subordinates to do what they should be doing.

Exercise 3. Find out your areas of strength and weakness

Score your performance out of ten for each item, then get members of your staff and your senior to score you for a selection of the items – they may see things differently.

Question	Self-rating	Staff rating	Senior rating
1 How much freedom of action do you allow your subordinates?			
2 Are you under pressure, unable to keep on top of the job?			
3 Do you keep subordinates informed about company policies?			
4 Do you adequately communicate the facts of changing situations to enable your subordinates to make good decisions?			
5 Is your superior prepared to encourage you to delegate by giving you added responsibility?			
6 Are you sufficiently courageous to risk subordinates making a mistake when it is you who may have to take the rap?			
7 Are you prepared to let others have a go, even if they don't do it your way?			
8 Your subordinates do the technical, routine and repetitive tasks: do you also give them the opportunity to be creative?			
9 Do you encourage subordinates to set their own work targets?			
10 Is it possible for your staff to monitor their own work progress?			
11 Are your subordinates encouraged to learn new skills or to improve their existing skills?			
12 Are your subordinates encouraged to take greater responsibility for their own work?			
13 Do you recognise the importance of delegating only within the range of competence of the individual?			
14 Do you accept your responsibility to develop subordinates to take on greater responsibility and do you act on it?			
15 Have you systematically identified the activities you wish to delegate in the interest of motivating your subordinates as well as your own time-effectiveness?			

16 Do you monitor the delegated task and give
    positive feedback on how it is being performed?
17 Do you accept that you remain accountable
    for all delegated activities?
18 Do you delegate some tasks simply because
    you dislike them?
19 Do you resist delegating some tasks because
    you enjoy them?
20 Do you properly reserve all decisions on policy
    to yourself or colleagues?
21 Have the responsibilities of your
    subordinates been clarified and communicated
    by means of detailed job descriptions?
22 Are individuals made aware of their
    opportunities for growth and development by
    means of regular performance appraisals?
23 Do you delegate the right to be wrong?
24 When dealing with questions, do you ask
    the individual how he/she would handle it?
25 Do you analyse bad decisions and learn
    from them?

Exercise 4.[2] Ask yourself which of these matters is managing the job or actually doing the job:

1 Calling a meeting to gain information from staff on how quality could be improved.
2 Reviewing appraisal records.
3 Signing an authorisation form for routine stationery re-stocking.
4 Lunching with a visitor from outside the organisation who is touring your facilities.
5 Working up a new system for decreasing nursing supplies.
6 Calling referees from a former job to verify employment dates on a job application.
7 Attending a routine but important meeting on recent PCT guidelines on reimbursement forms.

What did you think?

1 Managing – but ask an assistant to arrange meeting venue/times.
2 Managing – confidential information.
3 Doing – get someone else to sign up to a certain limit.
4 Managing/doing – a public relations exercise that could be given to someone to develop them. Depends on who the visitor is.
5 Doing.
6 Doing.
7 Doing – ask one of your staff to go for you and report back.

CHAPTER 10

Interviewing skills

Section 1 Selection, Counselling and Grievance Interviews

'Give every man thine ear, but few thy voice'

Polonius *(Hamlet)*

Almost as much time needs to go into preparing for interviews as the interview itself.

The people and interpersonal communication skills needed in all types of interview are:

- good listening
- active questioning
- summarising
- problem solving
- planning
- diagnostic
- evaluative
- reflective
- non-judgemental
- non-directive
- accepting.

This section on interviewing skills looks in more depth at when, where and how these skills can be both acquired and applied.

Developing listening skills

Listening well is difficult. Most adults retain only 25% of what they hear when they are not actively listening. This is because:

- we prejudge – we hold prior expectations of what the speaker is about to say
- our minds wander
- we fake attention
- noise, distractions, time pressure and our own internal thoughts may interfere.

Active listening is a physically demanding, conscious process of attending to what the speaker is saying. Active listening skills are needed for all people management tasks, but particularly during selection, counselling and grievance interviews.

How to develop listening skills.

- Remember we can listen, and process information, faster than we can speak.
- Eliminate distractions.
- Stop talking, don't interrupt.
- Relax, don't rush.
- Be alert to non-verbal cues.
- Empathise.
- Demonstrate understanding, paraphrase/summarise frequently.
- Use open-ended questions to clarify and understand.
- Use silence, don't be afraid of tension.
- Allow for reflection.

The selection interview

Selection interviewing is one of the most important jobs to be done in a practice, and time and energy need to be spent on both the preparation and conduct of the interview. For this you will need:

- interpersonal communication skills
- problem solving skills
- analytical skills
- planning skills.

What can help?

- Interview no more than four candidates, otherwise decision-making can be difficult.

- Note your personal prejudices and put them aside. Do you feel intimidated by the candidate? It is easy to be put off by those with good degrees if you haven't got one. Use your person specification as a guide.
- Standardise the interview and have a system for evaluation of results so as to avoid the risks of bias or the halo effect (the person reminds you of your mother/best friend/an irritating colleague).

Preparation

Preparation is crucial.

- Use an unbiased assessment method.
- Collect together all the information you require.
- Think about the interview plan (headings or areas needing discussion) and the environment.
- Organise the panel, giving each all the necessary documentation.
- Clarify any outstanding issues with the interview panel beforehand so you present a cohesive and united front. If you can offer incentives to attractive candidates discuss financial ceilings before your interviewee is present.

Environment

- Tailor your environment to the type of interview, but ensure it is relaxed and equal.
- Provide refreshments for the candidates.
- If there is a delay keep those waiting informed.
- Ensure that there are no interruptions while the interview is in progress. Allow the candidate to feel the focus of your attention.

Panel membership

- Aim for no more than three if possible; too large a group can be intimidating and unworkable for questioning.
- If a larger number is essential make certain that only two or three members hold the overall responsibility for questioning – others can act as observers and feed their questions into the panel beforehand.

Conduct of interview

The communication skills required here are informative, open and evaluative.

- Interviewing is a professional, not a personal, encounter.
- Show who is in charge – introduce yourself by name and function.
- Outline the conduct of the interview: 'We'll start by talking about yourself and your career then give you an opportunity to ask questions.'

- Do not allow the candidate to interview you, but respect that they need to find out about you as much as you do about them.
- Listen well.
- Write notes, which are essential as a record.
- Work towards helping the interviewee clarify the various options open to him or her.
- Be honest if there are any problem areas in the job.
- Summarise frequently, this helps to clarify ideas for all involved.
- Make a final summary where you confirm the areas covered during the interview.

Questioning structure

- Prepare and agree questioning with all the panel membership well in advance of the interviews.
- Aim to get the candidate to do the talking in a controlled way on topics under your direction.
- Keep your own questioning short, the candidate is there to shine not you.
- Start the conversation on an easy area where the interviewee can talk freely.
- Ask more probing questions once the candidate has settled.
- Aim for a non-directive style, diagnostic and reflective rather than interrogative, by using non-threatening questions and encouraging joint problem solving.
- Avoid leading questions where the expected answer rather than the true answer is revealed.
- Aim for continuity of questioning rather than disjointed hops from topic to topic.
- Use questions that are open-ended and that reflect back once the initial setting has been achieved.
- Reserve the first section for a consideration of the interviewee's employment background
- Ask open questions, e.g.
  - What did you dislike most about your previous job?
  - Of all the bosses you have had, which one did you like most/least and why?
  - If we asked your last boss about your work performance, what would they say?

The second stage could focus more on the job on offer, and how this person could satisfy the job requirements.

- Ask questions that relate to the person's past experience, e.g.
  - How do you think that your experience makes you a suitable candidate?

- This job has a commitment to working to deadlines. How do you feel about that and what is your experience of this?
- I see that you were on a working party to computerise your last organisation. What was your involvement and did you enjoy it?
- What do you feel has been your most successful achievement to date?
- Have you ever had a crisis at work and how did you deal with it? (Rather than what would you do if ...?)
- What do you feel you have done particularly well?

To complete

- Here is the chance for candidates to sell themselves. At the very least, expect some questions about the organisation and future prospects.
- Ask if there is anything else the candidate could tell you that may affect your decision.
- Ask if he/she would take the job if offered.
- Let the candidate know when they will be contacted.
- Don't be afraid not to appoint if unsure; you will undermine your own position far more by appointing someone ineffective or incompetent.

Follow-up

- Inform all applicants of your decision.
- Contact all interviewees as soon as possible after the interviews.
- Do not send out the rejection letters until the chosen candidate has accepted.
- Take up references before making an offer of employment.
- Contact a previous rather than present employer for a more honest assessment.
- Look at the implications behind statements such as 'Susan works well under close supervision' – what is not said in a reference is often more telling than what is.
- Arrange for the new member of staff to start and prepare your induction programme.

The counselling interview

It may fall to the person with a management role in the practice to offer a counselling interview to an employee whose personal problems are interfering with their ability to work at their best. Many employers are now using this opportunity to refer their employee to their own in-house or external counsellor supported by an occupational health scheme. Many more use the existing counselling skills of their GP colleagues. It is preferable to refer externally, as a clear boundary is created and the material remains confidential. Be wary of using your own GPs, as it is difficult to separate out the 'counsellor' and employer roles.

An external referral is without doubt the first choice for individuals displaying entrenched or severe distress. The counselling interview described below can be used for more minor problems, such as persistent lateness or an increase in errors. The manager's role in this instance is to clarify the reasons for the work-related difficulties, before deciding on a course of action.

The objective

The objective is to listen to and give advice on problems that may directly or indirectly affect the individual's work. Although person-centered counselling skills[1] are used, the person 'counselling' is not employed in a counselling role, but simply applying first line counselling **skills,** which are:

- empathic and supportive
- non-intrusive
- listening
- open questions
- reflective
- observational
- accepting and non-judgemental
- summarising.

The interviewer will direct or guide the interviewee, with an aim not to tell but to help the interviewee to solve or come to terms with the problems themselves. The skills used are taken from the humanistic school of counselling, taught originally by Carl Rogers. Rogers' core belief was that every human had within them the ability to see, and solve, their own dilemmas, without direct intervention and analysis from an outsider. Therefore, the counselling role is not to solve but to assist.

In humanistic counselling practice the counsellor adapts their way of working to suit or 'fit' the individual. The interviewer, in this instance, acts to provide a sense of:

- choice
- safety
- positive self-regard
- focus of evaluation
- congruence
- open presence
- encouragement
- ongoing commitment to the interviewee.

The interviewee, if given adequate time and space with which to explore their problem, will know when the work begins and ends, but the 'counsellor' provides a safe boundary through agreeing some core conditions of:

- time (length of session – when it begins and ends)
- length ('Shall we look at this together over the next few weeks, each Wednesday')
- confidentiality (what can be disclosed to a third person, when and under what circumstances).

Preparation

- Keep a record of specialists who could give help.
- Ensure privacy.
- Give adequate time.
- Check limits of own authority and ability.
- Look at individual's file.
- Plan approach according to the individual.

Applied skills

- Demonstrate understanding not sympathy.
- Ask open questions to encourage the interviewee to talk freely. ('Tell me some more about that', 'What happened then?', 'Why do you think that is?')
- Use closed questions when you are looking to get to the core of the problem, or close the interview. These questions require a one word or yes/no response only. ('Who do you feel able to ask for support?', 'When can you arrange that?')
- Reverse questions and statements to encourage the person to problem solve:
  Interviewee: 'The baby is keeping me awake night after night, and my memory seems to be going.'
  Interviewer: 'You feel exhausted and unable to cope as you used to.'
- Listen, observe and reflect back the interviewee's feelings, as you see them, and summarise for them. As an outsider, you are more able to do this. Note understated feelings particularly and draw these to the interviewee's attention:
  Interviewee: 'I wish that X could help with the extra work, but he can't, he's got his own job to do.'
  Interviewer: 'It sounds like you are disappointed and angry with X for not helping more.'
  Problem solve: How could we solve this? What will your next step be?
  Summarise with a positive conclusion and agreement as to future action.

Follow-up

* Arrange for future interviews to check developments.
* Carry out any action promised.

The grievance interview

The objective of a grievance interview is to enable a person to air a complaint, to discover the causes of dissatisfaction and, where possible, to remove them.

Preparation

* Find out as much about the grievance as possible – facts, attitudes, feelings.
* Consult other people for advice.
* Check the individual's file for any previous, similar, situations.
* Confirm own limits of authority.
* Check organisational policy and be clear about the organisation's grievance procedure.
* Allow for time and privacy.
* Find out if the individual is bringing a representative.

Skills

* Be calm but positive.
* Allow the grievant to 'let off steam first'.
* Check your mutual understanding of the exact situation and the facts.
* Listen carefully.
* Probe deeply.
* Do not belittle the issue or dismiss it.
* Finish with positive action for the future.
* Ascertain you both understand what happens next.

Follow-up

* Investigate facts and possible causes of action.
* Write notes.
* Follow-up interview.
* Take any agreed action.

Dealing with the chronic complainer

For some people nothing works, but a negative attitude prevails. If this is the case, rather than letting the employee have a contagious effect on the work group, positively confront them.

- Give them recognition for what they are doing well.
- Reassure and encourage them if they feel outdated or overwhelmed with new challenges.
- Accept their behaviour if it is not interfering with their performance.
- This complainer may be a spokesperson for the group. Check to see whether the complaint or ill feelings are more widely held, and follow up to correct.

Reference

1   Rogers C (1967) *On Becoming a Person*. Constable, London.

Section 2 Appraisals

In this section we will look at the sorts of communication skills required for appraisals. Good appraisers will also use the listening and counselling skills outlined in the previous section.

Clearly people achieve more when they are given adequate feedback on how they are performing, given clear attainable goals, and involvement in task setting. That said, the majority of managers do not like appraising staff and look for ways to avoid it. Do you:

- feel you have time to appraise staff?
- avoid giving constructive criticism?
- believe in self-appraisal?

Appraisals are another way of demonstrating that you believe in your staff. An appraisal is:

- a formal system for examining and building on your staff's strengths and minimising their weaknesses
- a space for staff to assess their own needs and areas of difficulty
- an opportunity to discuss potential.

Appraisals can highlight problems and improve communications. Appraisal is not:

- subjective
- ever attempted without the support and commitment of the whole management team
- telling staff what is going wrong
- a disciplinary interview
- applied on the basis of insufficient, inadequate or irrelevant information
- ever dishonest
- presented as fact instead of opinion
- an opportunity to re-emphasise past problems.

Do you:

- monitor staff performance?
- make informal judgements on behaviour and work performance on a daily basis?
- note positive, as well as negative, aspects of performance?
- hold the attitude that most people are well aware of their good and bad points, and will strive within a job to improve themselves?
- respond appropriately and instantly to unacceptable behaviours?
- set standards for the staff that make clear what is expected in terms of behaviour?
- have written examples of what occurs if the staff contract has been breached?

The appraisal interview

Everyone makes judgements about their staff, and the appraisal interview is an opportunity for both you and your staff to look at their job and their job performance in a more structured way. Ideally, it creates a space for staff to self-assess, to identify their own needs and areas of difficulty. The objective is not to tell the member of staff what is going wrong; it is not a disciplinary interview. The aim is to discuss potential for development, and subsequent training needs.

Monitor staff performance: all employers make informal judgements on their employees' behaviour and work performances. It is important to look at, and note, positive as well as negative aspects of their work on an ongoing basis.

Attitudes to colleagues and patients are transparent to the alert manager who spends time informally observing. Work well done needs to be praised. Thanks (verbal or written) are important if staff are expected to continue producing work of a high standard. Poor work or unacceptable behaviour needs challenging immediately.

- Set your standards for the staff and make clear at regular intervals what is expected of them in terms of behaviour.
- Anger directed at a patient should never be allowed to occur without some form of immediate staff counselling.
- Develop a written code and then you will be clearer when a breach of conduct occurs.

Prepare: it is the easiest thing in the world to avoid giving constructive criticism. If you allow staff the space to self-appraise and assess their own strengths and weaknesses, your own input may become unnecessary. Once they have identified a point to work on, it then becomes easier to offer pointers of your own.

Even if you work for a small organisation such as general practice, it is still important to prepare staff ahead. Inform them that you will be interviewing and when, and ask them to bring along their Personal Development Plan (PDP), where they consider their past performance, areas of achievement, and future training needs.

Communication skills during the interview: look together at ways of extending and improving work performance.

- Allow ample, uninterrupted and private time.
- Stress the two-way nature of the interview.
- Encourage staff to take the lead.
- Use open, reflective questioning so that the interviewee can expand on what they think.

- Ask for some specifics about how the job has gone that year.
- Make statements about performance after they have given their views.
- Add to, rather than submerge, their points.
- If the employee is closed to the idea of self-assessment, construct hypothetical situations so that they can assess their likely reaction, e.g.
  - How do you feel when angry, impatient people are on the telephone?
  - How do you react to the habitual attendee who you feel is wasting the doctor's time?
  - How do you feel when the doctor asks you to pass a message on that you know will be badly received?
  - Do you find it easy to delegate?
  - Do you find all the people who work here easy to get on with?
- Where poor performance is under scrutiny, emphasise 'how can we improve' rather than noting the problem.
- Summarise: listen and observe.
- Make a final summary emphasising conclusions and future action.

Follow-up:

- Complete an appraisal form that identifies current problems and targeted areas for action.
- Give a copy to the member of staff.
- Note areas that you have promised to investigate or change, and do so.
- Set a date, and make sure any action taken is also followed up.

Reward performance appropriately: if your staff are working particularly well, or producing work of a consistently high standard:

- notice it
- give verbal praise
- consider other pay or non-pay related benefits.

Everyone appreciates it when his or her work is noticed, and time spent in a good staff appraisal system is time well spent. In practices where there are formal or informal appraisal systems in use there tends to be less staff turnover and a happier working environment.

Giving constructive feedback

As managers, one part of our job is to give people positive and negative feedback so they can learn and develop their work skills. We also need to be able to express grievances to those who manage us; we can show others within the practice how best to do this assertively so that resentments and negative feelings do not fester.

Positive feedback

All too often we fail to give reward, or positive 'strokes' to people through embarrassment or awkwardness. People need to be told when they are doing splendidly; once good behaviour is reinforced it is more likely that it will be repeated.

- Be honest. Insincerity always negates the compliment. We often give insincere compliments as a response to being given one ourselves.
- Be specific. Avoid using vague statements like 'You were great/terrific'; these do convey a positive message but leave the other person unsure about what you mean. Try clarity:
  - I really admire the way you take so much time when you explain things to new staff. I can see you have a lot of patience.
  - That could have been embarrassing; I thought you diffused the situation very tactfully.
  - I'm very impressed by your ability to sit back and weigh up a situation before acting.
  - I admire the way you put the patients at their ease when they first come in.

Peer appraisal and appraisal for GPs

When was the last time anyone:

- asked you if you are happy in your job?
- gave you the space to tell them?

The ethos and culture of medicine makes peer appraisal difficult, but not impossible. The purpose of appraisal is not to undertake a disciplinary interview, but to work collaboratively to jointly review past performance, assess future potential, and find out what motivates and rewards the appraisee.

Whoever appraises should use assertive, counselling, problem solving and facilitation skills to be:

- fair and unbiased
- constructive and positive
- objective
- open and clear
- supportive yet challenging
- using evidence not anecdotes.

GP appraisals are therefore not hierarchically based, but seen as:

- developmental

- not performance managed
- focused on process, not clinical outcomes.

The personal development meeting, or appraisal, is primarily about the individual, their job and their development. The needs of the individual and the organisation they work within do not always coincide, so if conflict exists this should be explored. Those being appraised need to know what is expected of them, and obtain fair, constructive, objective and positive feedback on how they are performing. Appraisals should be conducted within an environment that is open, positive, supportive and developmental.

The appraisee should be given the opportunity to:

- engage in the discussion
- reflect on their own performance
- state their needs and expectations
- seek clarification
- set meaningful – subjective and objective – targets.

All judgements must be evidence-based and sourced, made on the basis of sound information.

What interpersonal and communication skills need to be appraised?
- Attitudes and personal effectiveness.
- Patient approach.
- Communication skills.
- Leadership skills.
- Contribution to the management process.
- Complaints.

You can address these challenges by developing your personal skills to learn how to deal with conflict, give constructive criticism, and learn to give and receive feedback. Your organisation can support you by:

- behaving in an open way
- developing strong and gifted teams
- reinforcing the concept of mutual support
- learning from its mistakes
- believing in the importance of service delivery
- training and developing staff
- being self-evaluative.

Introducing an appraisal system should be a positive, strengthening experience, which should build on the strengths of both the organisation and the individuals working within it. Everyone appreciates it when his or her good work is noticed, and time spent in a good staff appraisal system is time well spent. Praise leads to constructive self-analysis, which benefits the employer too. In practices where there are formal appraisal systems in use there tends to be less staff turnover and a happier working environment, which of course presents the practice in a better light to the outside world.

Section 3 Disciplining staff

Every organisation has staff that 'overstep the mark', and there comes a time when it becomes necessary to intervene. Most general practices avoid using the correct disciplinary procedures. Giving criticism is never easy, and if given badly it can lead to avoidable and expensive resignation. However, if one member of staff consistently makes mistakes and is not disciplined, the lack of boundaries and clarity can create a feeling of uncertainty amongst the other members of staff. They too may then work in an undisciplined way as they see the practice condoning bad behaviour without sanction. Here we examine some of the communication skills needed to make disciplining effective and easy.

Effective leaders:

- create clear guidelines, limits and boundaries
- are consistent and fair in their approach
- demonstrate that they understand the culture
- model mutual respect and clarity
- identify acceptable and unacceptable behaviour.

Giving criticism

The assertive person does not avoid expressing a grievance. Many working in general practice work under the assumption that it is easier to nurse grievances, but it is much wiser to clear the air. We all need to be told when we are doing something wrong in order that we may learn from the experience.

It **is** difficult to confront. It does seem much easier to let resentment build up, as we fear:

- hurting someone
- making a scene
- creating the wrong impression
- being disliked.

Badly given criticism can leave people feeling hurt or rejected, can feel like an attack, and can antagonise or confuse. We avoid giving criticism because we try to spare pain. In this way we protect people from their own feelings. But we do need to share our grievances before stored up resentments turn a small incident into a huge one. The aim is to communicate in a more civilised manner.

- Face the problem directly.
- Communicating vague resentments is passive and manipulative.
- Aggressive retorts leave people feeling hurt and angry.

- If you feel angry and critical, stop and think; the only valid reason for giving criticism is to help the other person grow, develop and learn from their mistakes.
- Allow people to accept or reject the criticism in their own way; they too are adults and must assume responsibility for dealing with the situation, and their feelings, as they wish. It is patronising to assume responsibility for your staff's emotional lives.

Giving constructive criticism

- Select your time and place wisely, a private room for example.
- Be specific: do not drop vague hints that you are irritated by, for example, poor time keeping, confront the issue: 'Helen, we feel frustrated when you are late, could you try to arrive by 4 o'clock next time?'
- Be prepared to compromise: 'If this time is difficult for you maybe we could think about starting the meeting later ...'
- Express how you feel about the behaviour, and the effect it has on you, the organisation or the patients. Take responsibility for your feelings: 'I feel angry when ...'
- Avoid direct attack and blame – whether in the form of 'You're so immature' or 'You should be more ...' This can be read as unsolicited, unwanted advice. Do not judge. Global or generalised statements about someone's behaviour are basically attacks on their personality. Again, state how you feel, specifically, about the one item of behaviour you want changed.
- Do not assume that you know what motivates other people, for you may be mistaken. Avoid analysis such as: 'You must have known how much that would hurt' – it is impossible to interpret other peoples' behaviour.
- Spell out the consequences of changed behaviour: 'I will feel much less strained if you could be on time.' If the change you anticipate or hope for does not come about, be prepared to ride the consequences. Remember that we can always change our behaviour, but we cannot expect others to change theirs, however much we want them too. You can ask, but you may not get what you want.
- View the other person as an equal. If you do take the initiative to confront, remember that you in turn may be confronted.
- Take responsibility: invariably, people are surprised, and often shocked, when you mention that part of their behaviour has had such an effect on you, so do take responsibility for not mentioning it before: 'I'm sorry that I didn't make myself clear before. I should have mentioned it, but I didn't feel able.'
- Invite criticism: 'Have I surprised/upset/angered you?'

- Empathise: understand the other person's position. Start with something on the lines of: 'I realise that what I have to say will be upsetting ...'
- Keep calm. Make sure that you keep your voice level and avoid using threatening gestures.
- Phrase positively: 'It would be better if you talked more loudly' gives someone the hope of being both better heard and better regarded if they make that change. Saying the same thing negatively: 'It would be better if you did not talk so quietly' can leave the person concentrating on their sense of failure rather than wanting to improve.
- End on a positive note: find a remark to balance the interaction. Give some indication that you value the other person and are not only seeing the negative: 'I'm grateful to you for listening' or 'I'm glad that we've aired this.' If you wish, you may like to add a positive statement about the other person: 'I do hope that my having said this will not adversely affect our relationship. I've always found you especially easy to talk to, and I do value the way we work so well together.' Or you may prefer to end the conversation with a positive consequence – something on the lines of: 'I'm glad that we've cleared the air. Now I feel that I'll be more relaxed in your company.'
- Be honest and true to yourself – mean what you say.

The disciplinary interview

Staff should be aware of any systems for discipline, and disciplinary procedures, in use. It is essential to have written job descriptions and contracts, so that staff will be aware when their work is not up to standard. It is then much easier to say, 'As you are aware, this is what we expected of you and you have broken your side of the deal.'

The objectives

The objective of a disciplinary interview is to inform of and correct mistakes or unwanted behaviour by helping the employee to improve – thus preventing the situation from arising again. It should not be viewed primarily as a means of imposing sanctions.

Interviewing for disciplinary problems

Disciplinary problems are to do with people's performance. Someone isn't doing what he or she ought to be doing. The aim is to improve performance in the future. This means that the whole emphasis must be on the future, looking forward rather than back. The style of the interview should be a problem-solving style – getting the facts, exchanging opinions, deciding action.

Basic guidelines

There are certain basic principles that will always apply to this kind of interview.

- You need to keep calm and control your temper even if you feel provoked. Remember the aim is to solve a problem; an aggressive attitude will never achieve this.
- You need to be seen to be taking the whole matter seriously.
- You need to focus on work performance, not personalities.
- You need to listen and let the interviewee do most of the talking. This is the only way to get the facts, get co-operation, and to prevent you from making a fool of yourself because you have not understood the problem.
- You need to aim for agreement on the problem and the action decided.

Specific techniques

Prepare
- Ensure that the interviewee clearly understands that it is a disciplinary interview, that they have received a formal warning and that the interview may form part of a dismissal procedure.
- They should be told in advance that they have the right to be accompanied by someone else if they wish.
- Plan a successful outcome (it will almost certainly be a change of some kind in the employee's behaviour).
- Plan the interview:
  - be clear about the reasons for seeing someone
  - have all the facts to hand
  - try not to pre-judge
  - plan approach according to the individual
  - consider your sanctions
  - know the procedure inside out
  - ensure privacy.

Opening
- Make sure you are both seated.
- Be clear: 'I thought we'd better have a talk because of your timekeeping in the last few weeks.'
- State the aim of the interview: 'I want us to get to the bottom of this matter and agree what to do about it.'

- Establish the objective of the interview.
- Ask the interviewee for their side of the story.
- Probe the information given:
  - did your employee know that an offence was being committed?
  - investigate the facts of the case thoroughly
  - allow the employee to put their case.
- Clarify expected standards of performance or organisational policy.

Manner
- Don't joke – this is a serious matter, show that you are taking it seriously.
- Keep calm – never allow yourself to lose your temper.
- Encourage frankness.
- Be firm, yet fair.
- Establish the facts; don't get bogged down in recriminations about the past.
- Commend good work and effort.
- Don't humiliate.

Listen
- Ask open-ended questions that cannot be answered just 'yes' or 'no' ('What effect do you think this has on other people?').
- Don't ask leading questions such as 'When are you going to stop disrupting other people's work?'
- Having asked a question, wait for an answer; don't worry about pauses.
- Pay attention to everything said; try to detect the feelings and attitudes behind the words.
- Encourage talking (nods, smiles, 'Hmm', 'Yes, I see').
- Show you have been listening; summarise the employee viewpoint and get them to agree that you've got it right.

Problem solving
- Draw the employee's attention to the fact that their action has led to difficulties for their colleagues; this may have more impact than an explanation that you or the practice has been let down.
- Help them to understand your problem.
- Get agreement on what the problem is.
- Keep the discussion to the point.
- Be prepared to amend your original view.
- Encourage the employee to suggest solutions.
- Discuss more than one possible solution.
- Make it clear that you cannot agree to grant special favours unless there are very special circumstances.
- Remind them of any laid-down procedures, such as the next stages in an appeals procedure.

Conclusion
- Agree on what you are both going to do.
- Agree a time-scale for follow-up.
- Tell the interviewee if you will be making any record of your interview or discussing the matter with anyone else.
- Check you have achieved your immediate aims.

Follow-up
- Write up notes immediately.
- Take any action you agreed on to help the individual, send copies to them.
- Look for ways to help the employee to avoid the same mistake in future.
- Decide on a reasonable length of time in which to improve.
- Clarify that any action has been understood.
- Fix a date to meet again.

Each disciplinary interview should be approached according to the stage of the procedure reached. Decide on the seriousness of the action. At the initial stages, an informal problem solving approach may be best, and considerate handling at this stage may prevent the matter from going any further.

In summary.[1]

- Discuss the performance, not the person.
- Use facts, not assumptions.
- Be objective, use records.
- Spell out limits and aims.
- Listen.
- Share the blame if necessary.
- Use mistakes to learn.
- Focus on the future, not the past.
- Find a better way.
- Affirm their ideas, compliment calm manners.
- Summarise.
- End on a high note.
- Follow up.

Problems in disciplinary interviews

The problem solving approach is the best for disciplinary interviews. Sometimes, however, it seems to be the last approach the interviewee wants. The interviewee tries to avoid the problem solving approach either by surrendering or attacking. If you are not to be deflected you need to understand these tactics and know how to avoid them. In all of these examples, **keep to the main purpose of the interview and don't be sidetracked.**[2]

- *The person who confesses everything.* They admit everything – including matters you didn't intend to discuss. The aim is to deflect your aim from the one aspect you wanted to discuss. **Action:** ignore the distractions; stick firmly to the point you want to discuss, e.g. 'It's that time-keeping problem that I particularly want to discuss at the moment.'
- *The one who cries.* They hope to embarrass the interviewer into backing down or abandoning the whole idea. **Action:** offer tissues. Wait. Then gently – but firmly – proceed as planned.
- *The person who claims to be in deep depression and full of problems* – to which hopefully, you won't add. **Action:** if depression is genuine, encourage referral. If not make it clear that you expect nothing exceptional, just the same standards as others and the same, presumably, as they formerly achieved.
- *The one who threatens their resignation.* An offer (threat?) usually accompanied by warnings of the difficulty of replacing the employee. **Action:** be wary; accepting their offer could lead you into a 'constructive dismissal'. Stick to the topic of the interview, e.g. 'We're not talking about resignation, we're trying to work out how to reduce the error rate on these accounts.'
- *The 'ambusher'* – lies in wait saying nothing until they have identified the weakness in your argument. Then they home in on it. **Action:** be sure of your facts before you start; ask questions to get them talking. If they do find a minor weakness, don't allow it to become the central issue, e.g. 'The exact time does not affect the main issue – your being late three days out of five'.
- *The 'shop-steward'.* Usually knows the rule book inside out and claims also to speak on behalf of the 'department'. **Action:** let them talk it out without being drawn into detailed arguments; keep the focus on their behaviour, e.g. 'Let's put what the department thinks to one side for the moment. What can you do to help solve this problem?'
- *The one who claims to be the injured, and innocent, party,* and can't believe they are being accused of doing something deliberately. **Action:** ignore the emotive words they use; don't start apologising for their deliberate misunderstanding of what you said: 'I just want to find out the reasons why the telephone was left unattended this morning.'
- *The buck passer* always has a hundred good reasons why it isn't their fault – someone else let them down etc. **Action:** be sure of your facts before you start.
- *The aggressor* believes attack is the best form of defence and will probably attack you verbally: your own work habits; your competence to discuss this with them, etc. **Action:** don't lose your temper – that's what they want; pin them down to what they are going to do towards solving the problem under discussion.

The termination interview

If a member of staff feels threatened by the disciplinary procedure, they may react proactively by handing in their notice. If this occurs, listen carefully to their grievance as it can tell you some important facts about your organisation and style of management. It may be that the employee has had inadequate training for the job, or has been poorly supervised. It certainly points to unsolved problems or unvoiced grievances, which may mean that in future you need to be more aware of undercurrents of stress at work and need to allow space for these to be voiced.

The objective is to:

* discover the real reason for them wanting to resign
* use what you have learnt to prevent others from leaving.

You may wish at this stage to persuade an individual to change his or her mind, but if you fail, wish them well in their choice as it is in your organisation's favour to secure employee goodwill.

Further help

Always seek legal advice before embarking on a disciplinary procedure. Investigate all the training options before considering dismissal. You may need to seek the advice of:

* your Union, professional support organisation or Industrial Relations Advisors
* The Advisory, Conciliation and Arbitration Service (see the ACAS Code of Practice on Disciplinary Practice and Procedures in Employment)
* your employing Trust personnel department.

References

1   Fred Pryor Seminars (1997) *How to Supervise People*. Pryor Resources Inc., Shawnee Mission Parkway, Kansas.
2   Sourced from Brighton College of Technology – *Supervisors' Manual* (1997).

Further reading

* Phillips A (2002) *Assertiveness and the Manager's Job*. Radcliffe Medical Press, Oxford.

CHAPTER 11

The learning organisation

'Tell me and I will forget; show me and I may remember; involve me and I will understand'

(Motto on Redzebra T Shirt)

In management terms, learning is important as it helps with:

- self development – we learn both skills and knowledge, and the social norms – how to be and do
- development of others – training develops potential
- the development of a learning culture – enabling more creative, innovative thought.

This chapter begins by discussing the importance of developing learning within your organisation, and examines some of the principles and methods of the different approaches to learning. It finishes by looking at some of the more advanced communication skills needed by a mentor or learning set advisor.

Within our rapidly changing work environment, for any organisation to be effective it needs to be a learning organisation. Such an organisation is characterised in part by curiosity, a hunger for new ideas, and an openness to thinking.[1]

Basic principles of learning:

- It is part of a continuous improvement.
- What is taught does not equal what is learned.
- We learn most from sources other than courses.
- Organisational and individual needs can be integrated.
- We need to own our own learning.
- Problems come before subjects or solutions.

In the same way we are motivated by different things, we all have different attitudes to, and ways of, learning. Managers need to consider some of the different motivations and styles of learning and ability amongst their staff.

- How can you best learn to support each individual's development?
- Are you aware of the different learning abilities and preferences amongst your staff?

A learning organisation continually transforms itself. Creativity is encouraged and results occur. Practices wishing to develop in this way must encourage and develop their staff's need and desire to learn. Good communicators do this by viewing staff as partners in the process.

Step 1: Understand some of the obstacles to learning

> **Make a list of those things you see as preventing learning in your practice.**
>
>
> Lack of funding
>
> Lack of understanding and unwillingness to learn about difference
>
> Fear of change, failure   Lack of time
>

Step 2: Identify learning needs

What are your own and staff training needs? Encourage everyone to write a learning plan for his or her personal development folder. This requires an honest and valuable analysis of their present position and how that position was reached. It identifies the progress required and analyses what must be achieved to obtain that progress.

- Where have you been?
- Where are you now? Current knowledge, opportunities.
- Where do you want to get to?
- How will you get there?
- How will you know when you've arrived? (Goals are sharpened when the learner has to say how the learning will be measured.)

Step 3: Understand preferred learning styles

Developing organisations will be interested in adopting new, more modern, training and development methods, where the learner constructs their own learning and therefore actively participates in the process. Learning then is more complete, and more likely to fix. The teacher's role is to facilitate, mentor, assist and empower, not to impart knowledge.

We all have a preferred learning style. Over the years, we develop learning habits that help us benefit more from some experiences than others. If you are able to pinpoint your own learning preferences you will be in a better position to select the learning experiences that best suit your style. Researchers have classified certain types of learner[2]:

- The activist who learns by doing.
- The pragmatist who learns best when the practical application is obvious.
- The theorist who needs to understand the fundamental principles.
- The reflector who learns by thinking about things.

The new ways of learning are not passive, but encourage people to develop:

- self-awareness
- analytical thinking
- problem solving abilities
- further understanding of group processes and individual behaviour.

Practices are being asked, in developing Personal Learning Plans (PLP) and Professional Practice Development Plans (PPDP) to look beyond their traditional learning routes to meet new government expectations. They will need to demonstrate that they are broadening and developing their staff. Self-managed learning is one way of meeting this need.

What is self-managed learning?

One method of self-managed learning is to attend a **learning set**. Here, colleagues who share a common purpose meet to:

- share problems and ideas
- reflect on ways of managing difficult or new situations.

Learning sets:

- are a training method
- are where each group member has protected time to speak and be actively listened to
- are facilitated externally.

Groups can learn to facilitate themselves, to deal openly with any conflicts or difficulties that arise. It is through dealing with the difficulties that most of the learning occurs.

Learning sets help best:

- when working on real problems, engaging with others in mutual support and challenge

- when the focus is on personal development. When using protected time within the group to focus on difficult personal issues, usually around communication or work relationship difficulties, change can occur. The role of other group members is to listen, then comment, support, and maybe point in the right direction.
- For independent study – where you plan your own learning through a 'learning contract'.

Self-managed learning aims to create a situation where learning is owned by the individual and at the same time is closely integrated with organisational need.[3] It is an approach which is overtaking older methods such as lectures, tutoring and examinations, where the aim is to obtain paper qualifications. It is a dynamic, inspirational and creative way of learning; the learning occurs through applying new learned behaviour and methods to a working situation. It is a method of learning for anyone but is especially useful to those who need to develop good people skills and learn how to deal with conflict.

- It is *strategic*: this is not a shortsighted approach, e.g. about an exam to pass.
- It is *structured*: it operates within the real constraints of organisational life, working within resource and policy limits.
- It is *self-managed*: the learning occurs through interactions with others; there is joint problem solving, with greater flexibility and speed of response.
- *Shared*: through connections with others and thus integrated with organisational need.
- *Supported*: one support structure is the 'learning set' – a group of five or six learners who meet regularly, without interruptions to the working schedule.
- *Syllabus free*: the learning is driven by the real needs of the individuals and their organisation.
- *Stretching*: there is a requirement to set goals and meet them, having to meet and discuss progress with colleagues means you have to keep to your agreed plan.

The advantages of self-managed learning

- Finding more innovative solutions to problems.
- Learning is disseminated more widely.
- The benefits of networking: finding other people support you through change.
- Learning to support and challenge behaviour appropriately; actively listening, being more honest and open – and taking these skills back to the organisations.
- The facilitation skills can be learned and extended to others.
- Progress may be made on problems to which there may have been no clear solutions before.

- Participants are more open to further self-development.
- The focus is on approaching and dealing with practical problems, not on theory.
- Risk is soon regarded as a developmental and acceptable tool.
- People adapt the process to suit their own needs.
- Real issues are addressed, there is practical, immediate application of the learning.
- Individuals identify their own needs and arrive at their own solutions.

Leaders and supervisors within the practice benefit hugely from this sort of learning, and the self-reflection that occurs supports PDPs.

Learning sets demand peer group interaction, and ask that each participant is given equal time within the group. The person receiving the focus of attention learns, and evaluates, for themselves. There is a shift in his or her ideas in relation to the issue. The process can be supportive but challenging. For this to occur one needs:

- a facilitator who assists the group in making the most of the experience
- assessment: members need to provide explicit evidence for the ways they have changed once the set has completed
- group evaluation: the group evaluates the value of the course at its completion
- mentor: one from within the working environment, and one from outside the organisation, to provide development support.

The role of the mentor is to assist and support individuals through their change and development.

Seek out someone with good counselling skills who is able to:[4]

- share, not judge
- be honest and allow vulnerability
- retain confidentiality
- have credibility
- teach, and challenge, well
- sponsor
- network.

The role of the facilitator or set advisor is to:

- provide the framework
- move the group towards learning
- summarise
- note group dynamics
- intervene if needed.

For this they need to be able to:

- provide a positive, unconditional attitude
- see that everyone in the group is an individual, an exception, to be valued
- tolerate uncertainty
- have a secure sense of self
- have good interpersonal, listening and questioning skills
- hold an individual and group focus
- be non-judgemental.

(*See* also Chapter 12, Teaching and presentation skills.)

The set advisor will ask open-ended questions of their group – 'how' not 'why'. The 'why' encourages more rational, linear, thought, not creative questioning. They are an active participant in the group meeting, and their role is not to lead the meeting but to facilitate.

Guidelines for set meetings

Each individual has to:

- accept responsibility for their own learning
- collaborate with others in their learning
- learn not to take over
- listen actively
- be honest – say if you don't follow or understand, don't pretend
- accept other people's diversity and difference
- be sensitive to other's needs
- act confidentially – unless general decisions need to be communicated outside the group
- speak for themselves without generalising
- not speak, if it seems appropriate.

Set advisors are bound by the same rules, and have equal trouble following them!

Overcoming problems

- Selling the idea of set meetings to GPs can be especially difficult – medicine and GP training is very objective. Some older doctors are sometimes unhappy with 'soft' learning approaches; younger GPs can be more open and receptive to new methods. Older style training often carries objective knowledge gain; with self-managed learning the benefits are 'felt' and very subjective.
- You need time out from your work to attend the set. Some of your colleagues may be very focused on the here and now; they work reactively

and sometimes their investment in time out for training can be hard to secure – they want you in the practice, focusing on the job in hand! Be clear about your learning objectives, and be prepared to demonstrate by illustrating new ways you have of managing difficult situations.

- Meetings need to be well handled so they do not become unfocused.
- Set advising is challenging, and training as an advisor needs resourcing well.
- Programmes must be designed to suit the organisation and its culture.
- Some people find self-managed learning difficult:
  - they feel that others should be responsible for their development
  - they are unable to work successfully as part of a group
  - they believe they have nothing to learn about anything.

Developing advanced communication skills

Group facilitation requires huge skill. You need to develop awareness of your own responses, conscious and unconscious, so you can identify which learning style you are promoting. This requires learning how to develop a more rounded communication style and awareness. Here is a list of examples.

Behaviour	Why?
Asking why	Problem solving/analytical response
Suggesting issues are raised in the set, reminding members it is not your job to act on behalf of the set	Moderately confronting; promoting personal and group responsibility
Confirming that problems will arise between people in a group and asking how they might resolve it	Supportive; less confronting
Emphasising choice, helping individuals explore the choices open to them	Low direction; analytical
Pointing out that what happens in a set can exemplify problems that can occur elsewhere, and that resolving such problems can be a useful part of the person's learning	Raising process issues
Do nothing and wait and see if X does anything	Low intervention style; low confronting; low directiveness
Ask X if Y's ideas are useful	Questioning style; analytical – deflecting to problem owner and re-establishing his/her ownership

continued overleaf

Behaviour	Why?
Thank Y for his/her comments and ask if he/she thinks what he/she is doing is useful for X	Fairly high confronting; tackling Y as 'the problem'
Stop the set process, suggest a consideration of the purpose of the set – is it there to offer solutions?	Analytical; group process orientated; acting as referee; set adviser as guardian of the group process; moderately confronting
Tell X he/she is looking uncomfortable and ask the reasons	Supportive
Making physical contact (touch on the arm or shoulder)	Modelling set norms (enabling)
Let a set member know verbally that it is OK to cry	Permission giving, supportive; establishing/confirming set norms (intervening)
Say nothing, but demonstrate non-verbally (posture, movement pattern, etc.) to the rest of the set that you are comfortable with what is happening	Low intervention style: modelling; giving set responsibility to handle their problems
Ask upset member what s/he wants right now (e.g. does s/he want support from the set?)	Permission giving; problem solving
Do nothing	Low intervention style; low executive function; low leadership mode
Confront the set with the problem without suggesting a solution	Process intervention; not heavily confronting
Suggest that the set might consider some options for better timetabling, e.g. fixing a time for each person	Problem solving; propose/consult level of directiveness; potential structuring intervention
Telling the set how you feel	Openness; modelling expression of feeling
Ask the person who has gone last how they feel about having little time	Analytical; process intervention (but focused at individual level)
Do nothing and let the set sort it out	Low intervention style; low direction, low structuring, low leadership
Assist people to come to a consensus decision, e.g. ask how long the set is prepared to wait for a late arrival	Problem solving; low confronting, questioning mode plus group process intervention
Wait until the person arrives and then confront the set about the need to resolve the problem, e.g. find out reasons for the person's lateness; agree on how long the set will wait for late arrivals, etc.	Moderately confronting, structuring, non-leadership mode

Notes on the role of the set advisor

- The set is to help people to learn – it is not a therapy group.
- Its efficacy is to be judged by whether people learn (or not). Good set advising is related to how well you assist others to learn, and learn yourself.
- The set will not always be a comfortable place to be.
- Each person is responsible for his or her own learning – you are responsible to them to assist as appropriate.
- Support 'being'.
- Challenge behaviour ('doing').
- Check any question: is what I am about to ask going to assist the other person's learning?
- Helping members to help each other can be a key need. This may mean encouraging people to challenge each other, especially through questioning each other.
- People may need encouragement to ask for help
- Assume set members are sensible people who do want to learn to be better – even if the evidence appears to be to the contrary!
- Get members to take appropriate responsibility, e.g. for fixing venues, for asking for what they want.
- Model appropriate behaviour, but do not aim to be perfect – be a human being.
- Trust cannot be artificially created – you have to be genuine and sincere in what you do.
- You can assist people with activity outside the set, e.g. by pointing them to resources that they may not know about.
- Avoid: 'if I were you I would ...'. You are not the other person and never can be.
- Maintain the principles of the programme – you can't police people but you can confront them if they seem to have trouble 'playing by the rules'.
- Allow the group to handle issues for itself – but if no one does pick up on an issue you have a role in pointing it out.
- At the start of a set you need to put energy into learning about the set members. You can only help them learn if you have first learned from them.
- Primary feedback – the evidence of your eyes and ears – is usually more reliable than secondary feedback (comments on what has happened).
- Establish at the start that you are a neutral person who does not have a vested interest in the set's work.
- In preparing for a set meeting it can be useful both to prepare 'mechanically', i.e. plan how to get to the meeting or re-read contracts, and to prepare 'mentally', e.g. by thinking about each set member as a person, visualising them, etc.

- Even if you did little or nothing in a set, your role would be valuable.
- If you genuinely care about helping set members to learn, what you do is probably right.

References

1   Oldham J (2001) Key GP advisor says patients welcome advanced access. *Pulse*. **July 28**: 16.

2   Honey P (1994) Styles of learning. In: A Mumford (ed.) *Handbook of Management Development* (4e). Gower, London.

3   Morton-Cooper A and Palmer A (eds) (1999) *Mentoring and Preceptorship* (2e). Blackwell Science, Oxford.

4   Sourced from Crunningham I (1995) *Strategic Developments* and Sang B, Set Advisor to East Sussex NHS Fund Managers (1996/7).

Further reading

- McGill I and Beaty L (1992) *Action Learning*. Kogan Page, London.

CHAPTER 12

Teaching and presentation skills

Many primary care managers have a teaching or training role; many others are expected to give presentations as part of their job. The guidelines given here will assist with both. Good teaching and leading are very similar and there are similar principles to consider.[1] Both:

- recognise that every student/staff member is a unique, valued individual
- need to be able to command the respect of their charges, not only by their knowledge of what they teach but their ability to make it interesting
- need to be curious about what their students say and think
- assess their student's performance, reinforce the good work, and correct the bad
- are role-models
- demonstrate a participative management style
- have enthusiasm, commitment and ambition
- are effective communicators
- have integrity
- demonstrate that intensity coupled with commitment is powerful and magnetic
- stretch and challenge their students.

When training, remember that each individual has their own preferred learning style, and may learn best through doing (an active learner), reflecting, theorising or applying to a practical situation (pragmatist). Try to cater for all styles. When you are teaching, mix your mediums by using:

- text, pictures and concepts
- overheads, handouts, slides
- individual and group work
- problem solving and analysing
- discussion and direct teaching
- talking and listening

- visual images and diagrams
- replica objects
- tricks, humour, quizzes, e.g. members of the class participating in a body sculpture to model the different functions.

What levels of ability do you assume when working with, training or developing your staff? How do you ask for information? Every individual has communication strengths and weaknesses, and it is your role to elicit the best from your staff.

Do you:

- use open-ended or closed questions?
- use multiple choice?
- give a choice of written or verbal feedback?

For example, if you invite staff to write a short paragraph on their views of their work, this anticipates and demands a formal response that could intimidate those who are not familiar with a more formal, educated use of language and 'having to write too much'. Alternate your style, try check lists with yes/no answers to performance criteria.

Long-term teaching tips
Some principles

- The self-esteem of the learner underlies all learning. Build in reward and reinforcement systems.
- Some people have had difficult learning experiences and so have induced learner anxiety – be awake to this.
- Apply your messages consistently. Your expectations will be passed on consciously and unconsciously.
- Use positive, affirming language.
- Prepare.
- Start and end strictly on time.
- Corrections must be constructive and confidence-building rather than confidence-sapping.
- Remember students' perceptions are the reality. Stop talking – start listening.
- Be reliable, responsive, assuring, empathetic.
- Under-promise and over-deliver.
- Lead people do not manage them.
- Explore, experiment. Fail and try again. Build in open-mindedness, receptivity and sense of exploration to learn.

The trainer's maxim.

- Tell them what you are going to tell them.
- Tell them.
- Tell them what you have just told them.

- Advise learners beforehand of topics or issues, which will be covered – visually map them out.
- Make reference to the different points on the map as the time progresses – build a sense of a journey with an ultimate destination.
- Encourage some advance thinking on, or related to, each topic or issue as it comes up. Have learners work in pairs to collect all they know about a topic before formal teaching about that topic begins.
- Give the Big Picture first – describe the learning that will take place and the learning outcomes. Outline the learning outcomes: 'By the end of this session you will ...'.
- Encourage learners to link the session outcomes to their own learning goals.

Some teaching methods

- Break the topic into chunks. The most items of information an individual readily remembers is seven. Seven plus or minus two is often quoted as the optimum.
- Visual display of the subject material around the classroom improves the long-term learning by 90%.
- Use individuals who have achieved in their field to provide positive role models.
- Introduce a complex topic and then return to it, gradually building up the work on that topic. This allows the unconscious mind to be processing the new information: sorting, selecting and connecting.
- Provide opportunities for students to demonstrate the new knowledge.
- Build in a review – 80% of new knowledge is lost within 24 hours without some sort of review. Review the content of lessons at the end of each, and before beginning a new topic. Encourage review homeworks using memory maps.
- Memory maps for note taking: use colour, bold images and space on the page for learners to build up their own unique way of making sense of the material.

Presentation skills

The skills of a good presenter differ from those of a facilitator. Here, the communication is mainly one-way.

Making a presentation to your colleagues may not rate as highly on the terror scale as, say, addressing a conference, but few people feel entirely comfortable at the prospect and even fewer actually enjoy it. The reason is simple – fear. Fear of humiliation, failure, embarrassment, loss of self-esteem and dignity. Even the most experienced speakers feel the symptoms of fear before and during a presentation.

The key to success is to use the adrenaline that fear produces. Harness its energy to help you perform well. Allow yourself ten minutes and try this exercise:

Make a list of the types of presentations you have to do as part of your job.

- Meetings with a few staff and colleagues?
- A full practice meeting?
- A report to your local group of colleagues/ board members?
- A conference?

Think back to one presentation that went really well and one you feel could have been done better.

- From your recollections, identify your strengths and the areas in which you need to improve.
- Identifying your fears and thinking carefully about your strengths and weaknesses are the first steps in learning how to make them more effective.

Presentation fears

- What is causing the nervousness?
- How can you deal with the symptoms?

- What is it about the topic that bothers you?
    - You don't know where to start?
    - How to string the ideas together?
    - What are your fantasies about the audience?

See the Appendix for some solutions to these common fears about presenting.

- The fear of drying up.
- Forgetting what comes next.
- Your fear of an expert in the audience.
- You fear you may leave out an important point.
- There may be an awkward customer in the audience.
- Being asked a question that you can't answer.
- Fear of your own voice.
- Not wanting to let the audience down.
- Feeling too shy, or uncertain of your performance.

Pinpoint the fear then it will be tangible, and therefore easier to deal with. Don't generalise: 'I couldn't talk about anything for more than two minutes' – re-word to: 'I couldn't talk for more than two minutes about *this topic* to *that audience*'.

The presentation

Prepare
- Go to the location beforehand. Note the seating arrangements and the time you are allocated.
- Select a medium that suits the audience size.
- Complete your preparations at least 24 hours in advance. Do not under-estimate the time needed for word-processing, photocopying, binding etc.
- Do not economise falsely. Prepare copies for all, plus some spares.
- If you are anxious, never attempt a day's work first and arrive tired, stressed and hungry.
- Find out about your audience: their interest, level of expertise and motivation.
    - How many people will there be?
    - What are they expecting from your presentation?
    - What do you want to achieve?
    - Are you aiming to inform or persuade?
    - Can you discuss what you want to say with some of the people attending before you finalise your presentation?
    - How interested is your audience likely to be in the subject?
    - What level of knowledge will they have about it?
    - Will they be familiar with any technical language or jargon?

- Will they have any preconceptions or misconceptions about the subject?
- How might they use what you have to say?
- Always have notes, with key phrases and subject headings.
- Memorise your introduction.
- Rehearse.

Structure
- Preface – opening courtesies, the topic, purpose, duration and shape.
- Introduce self – seek common ground, state your history, why you are the best person to speak.
- Give a brief outline of the present situation, why the need for change etc.
- Look at the principal alternatives your audience will want to consider.

Ending
- Summary of salient facts/arguments/key visuals.
- Propose the recommended course of action.
- Admit limitations of proposals, and then make persuasive points.
- Set target dates etc.
- Description of supporting literature to be distributed.
- Thank the audience for their attention.
- Invite questions (if appropriate).

Afterwards
- Discuss with colleague for reaction.
- Think about follow-up.

Presentation techniques
- Don't try to cram everything you know on the subject into your talk.
- Select the main points and include such detail as your audience is able to absorb.
- Link your main points together to produce a cohesive argument.

Delivery
- Decide the most appropriate form and level of language to use.
- Choose the least stressful method. If giving a conference paper, speak from a prepared manuscript.
- Help people to follow the flow of your argument by giving signposts, indicating the number of points you wish to address and reiterating them at appropriate junctures ('The second point I want to make is ...').
- If asked to think on your feet: don't panic, don't ramble, don't undermine yourself by saying, 'You will have to excuse my mistakes because I haven't had time to prepare anything on that topic' (they already know that).

Communication

Remember the importance of first impressions.

- Show enthusiasm.
- Make and maintain eye contact.
- Smile and try to look relaxed.
- Act confidently and your audience will believe that you are confident.
- Project your voice to the furthest edge of the audience.
- Speak clearly at a conversational speed.
- Try not to mumble or use a monotone delivery.
- Look at the audience – all of them. Control them by maintaining eye contact and responding to any signs of puzzlement or boredom.
- Don't bury your head in your notes or use 'fillers' such as 'er', 'um', 'right', 'you know'. Use pauses instead – they don't seem half as long to an audience as they do to you.
- Avoid unnecessary pacing around, fiddling or gesturing.
- Make sure you keep an eye on the time so your last points are not rushed.
- Finish as enthusiastically as you began.

Language

- Use short words/short sentences.
- Use active verbs – concrete nouns.
- Illustrate general statements with specific examples.
- Only use technical terms to an audience familiar with them.
- Use your own words.
- Avoid or explain jargon.
- Signpost and paragraph the presentation.
- Keep your voice up at the end of sentences.

Content

- What are the main points you need to make to get your message across?
- What would be the most informative and interesting title for your presentation?
- Write down how you want to influence your audience; this acts as a constant reminder of what you need to achieve and reduces a complex message to manageable chunks.
- Check that you are not changing the message to fit the slide!
- The structure may not suit your audience, and the audience is more important than the show.
- Choose three or four main points which interest your audience, and three or four secondary points for each one.
- Select a natural order, e.g. problem followed by solution, question followed by answer, need followed by fulfilment.

Dealing with difficult questions

- Quell your own emotional response.
- Make any objectives specific.
- Do not bluff or make excuses.
- Congratulate questioner and explain why not included, e.g. too technical for some.
- Defer to the question area of expertise, perhaps ask for views.
- Ask for more facts.
- Open the questions to the group.
- Explore the questions, ask questioner to elaborate and refine.
- Answer the questions.
- Admit ignorance, promise to find out.
- Defer to deal with matter privately at greater length later.
- Refer to an expert colleague (if available).
- Ask the questioner to answer their own question.
- Ask others in the group to answer the question.
- Have a good discussion.

Methods of presentation

These influence our thinking, understanding and interpretation of material.

- Would it be helpful to give the audience any information in advance, such as statistics?
- Would visual aids, such as slides or a laptop presentation, clarify important points and aid understanding?
- Take summary copies of your paper for distribution after the presentation.
- Convert statistics into charts and graphs wherever possible.
- Relegate detail to supporting documents.

When using text:

- use phrases, not single words or sentences
- keep lists parallel and in order
- use a mixture of upper and lower case type
- highlight the most important messages
- be consistent.

When using graphics:

- use one message per chart
- use action headings
- eliminate unnecessary links
- use highlighting to focus attention
- use histograms for looking at the frequency of occurrence
- use pie charts to compare the contribution of each value to a total
- use bar charts to compare across categories.

Some useful statistical terms in this context are:

- mean – the average
- mode – the most frequently occurring item or number
- median – the mid point in a distribution curve
- standard deviation – how the figures shown deviate from the expected normal probability of occurrence.

When using concepts:

- use analogies that are meaningful to the audience
- use shapes and pictures to show relationships
- make your visualisation match your words.

Making successful presentations
- Research and organise your material in advance.
- Learn as much as you can about the people in your audience.
- Use video or audio aids to hold attention and increase understanding.
- Prepare notes – but don't read all the time.
- Rehearse.
- Anticipate possible questions and prepare your answers.

If you are expected to give presentations as part of your job, use these guidelines to assist.

Use the principles of good communication to underpin all your behaviour at work, and you will begin to see demonstrable benefits in your relationships with staff, and your organisation. To recap, effective leaders are good communicators.

Effective leaders:

- listen
- are honest and open
- recognise everyone as a unique, valued individual
- remain awake, open and curious to the world around them
- understand the need for change
- have integrity, enthusiasm, commitment and ambition
- are role models for a participative management style
- stretch, challenge and develop others through good leadership, consultation and delegation
- reinforce the good, and support people in their mistakes.

Intensity coupled with commitment is powerful and magnetic. Demonstrate your new communication principles and command respect not only through what you teach but in your ability to make it interesting.

Use your new interpersonal communication skills in teaching, managing and leading. Become a more effective speaker and listener which will enable you to respond skillfully and sensitively to any modern healthcare challenge.

References

1   Sourced from Conway JK (1992) *Strategic Objectives for Learning*.

2   Sourced from *Examining the Fear of Carrying out a Presentation*. David Salomon's Centre, Kent Health Service Management Module, Cert Management, 1997.

Further reading

- Martin V (2000) Present tense. *Practice Manager*. **October**: 37–8.
- Smith A (1996) *Twenty-one Ways to Improve Learning*. Accelerated Learning, Network Educational Press.

Appendix

Some solutions to common fears about presenting[2]
The fear of drying up.

- Accept this could happen and ask yourself: 'what will I do when I dry up?'
- Do not hide the fact by apologising or blustering.
- Accept it has happened and get back on track and know that once you get going again all will be well.
- Fall back on a predetermined routine, which manages the temporary crisis.

Forgetting what comes next.

- Look at your notes. Your audience expects this, and may be reassured that you are taking care to check things.
- As long as you remember the idea or the concept you want to cover, then you can express the same idea in different words; ideas are more important than the words.
- Take your time. Adrenaline will be pumping around your system and one of the effects of adrenaline is that it seems to expand time – seconds can seem like minutes. The silence that falls when you stop speaking will only seem huge to you.
- Remember, when you are in an audience, you are quite happy to wait for, and work at, the presenter's pace, so don't let silence fluster you.

If there is an expert in the audience.

- Remember, they have not been asked to talk, you have.
- Know your audience, and what you are trying to achieve.
- Treat the specialist as a resource not a threat and enlist their help at the appropriate time.
- Ask them a direct question, listen carefully to the answer, summarise the answer with them, thank them for their help and then carry on with the next point.
- Remember you start with the advantage of being the presenter, so everyone – including the specialists – will expect you to set the pace.
- Take the lead, otherwise you unsettle and unnerve the audience.
- Do not antagonise the specialists by blustering to show that you know more than they do.

You may leave out an important point.

- Does it matter? Was it essential to your audience's understanding of the topic?
- If you are particularly forgetful, highlight and enlarge your text. Use cards.

There may be an awkward customer in the audience.

- Learn how to deal with difficult people.
- If they challenge your position, or are disruptive, remember that their problems and inadequacies have nothing to do with you, or your own feelings of insecurity.
- The chances of you meeting someone who has deliberately set out to destroy your talk are very slight.

You may get asked a question that you can't answer.

- Research your topic thoroughly.
- If the question is about an obscure point of detail, or you don't know, say 'I don't know. That point has never occurred to me before. Why do you ask?' Don't try to bluff it out.
- Decide if continuing with the point will contribute to your talk or detract from it.
- Ask yourself if it is reasonable to have all the answers to every conceivable question.
- If the point is worth pursuing, promise to look for the answer after the session has finished.

Fear of your own voice.

- Accent adds colour, interest and music to the words.
- Accents rarely detract from a presentation.
- Never try to hide your accent, or you could end up sounding ridiculous.

You fear letting the audience down.

- Remain concerned about the well-being of your audience, and then you are less likely to let them down.
- Learn about your audience and be clear about your objectives.

You feel you are too shy.

- Think about what your audience needs rather than what might or might not happen to you. Their needs are paramount.
- The fact that you are the speaker means that you start your presentation with a good measure of credibility.
- You may feel shy, but if you do your job properly you won't look it.

You feel you don't have the gift of the gab.

- Your presentation should not consist of aimless chatter, it should set out to achieve a clear purpose.
- You will need a reasoned, disciplined and objective approach.
- Some people adopt such an approach quite naturally, but the rest of us have to learn the techniques.

You've talked before, and felt it was unsuccessful.

- Then you know where you made the mistakes – where you meant to say things and forgot; the fact that you ran out of time; the examples you didn't quote. The audience would not have known any of these things.

Index